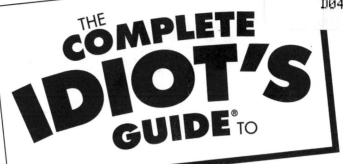

THE
**COMPLETE
IDIOT'S
GUIDE®** TO

Dairy-Free Eating

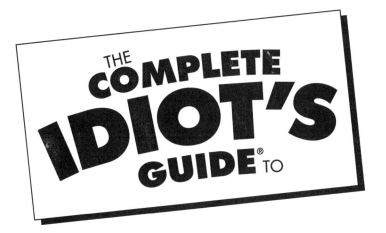

THE COMPLETE IDIOT'S GUIDE® TO

Dairy-Free Eating

by Scott H. Sicherer, M.D., and Liz Scott

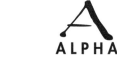

ALPHA

A member of Penguin Group (USA) Inc.

To my patients and everyone living milk free, with the sincerest hope that the advice and delicious recipes in this book will make living with this allergy easier; and to my wife, Mati, and children, Andrew, Cassaddee, Maya, Sydney, and Zachary, for their love and support. —Scott

To my family and friends whose support is indispensible. And of course, to Baby. —Liz

ALPHA BOOKS

Published by the Penguin Group

Penguin Group (USA) Inc., 375 Hudson Street, New York, New York 10014, USA

Penguin Group (Canada), 90 Eglinton Avenue East, Suite 700, Toronto, Ontario M4P 2Y3, Canada (a division of Pearson Penguin Canada Inc.)

Penguin Books Ltd., 80 Strand, London WC2R 0RL, England

Penguin Ireland, 25 St. Stephen's Green, Dublin 2, Ireland (a division of Penguin Books Ltd.)

Penguin Group (Australia), 250 Camberwell Road, Camberwell, Victoria 3124, Australia (a division of Pearson Australia Group Pty. Ltd.)

Penguin Books India Pvt. Ltd., 11 Community Centre, Panchsheel Park, New Delhi—110 017, India

Penguin Group (NZ), 67 Apollo Drive, Rosedale, North Shore, Auckland 1311, New Zealand (a division of Pearson New Zealand Ltd.)

Penguin Books (South Africa) (Pty.) Ltd., 24 Sturdee Avenue, Rosebank, Johannesburg 2196, South Africa

Penguin Books Ltd., Registered Offices: 80 Strand, London WC2R 0RL, England

International Standard Book Number: 978-1-59257-913-6
Library of Congress Catalog Card Number: 2009924906

11   10   09   8   7   6   5   4   3   2   1

Interpretation of the printing code: The rightmost number of the first series of numbers is the year of the book's printing; the rightmost number of the second series of numbers is the number of the book's printing. For example, a printing code of 09-1 shows that the first printing occurred in 2009.

Printed in the United States of America

Note: This publication contains the opinions and ideas of its authors. It is intended to provide helpful and informative material on the subject matter covered. It is sold with the understanding that the authors and publisher are not engaged in rendering professional services in the book. If the reader requires personal assistance or advice, a competent professional should be consulted.

The authors and publisher specifically disclaim any responsibility for any liability, loss, or risk, personal or otherwise, which is incurred as a consequence, directly or indirectly, of the use and application of any of the contents of this book.

Most Alpha books are available at special quantity discounts for bulk purchases for sales promotions, premiums, fundraising, or educational use. Special books, or book excerpts, can also be created to fit specific needs.

For details, write: Special Markets, Alpha Books, 375 Hudson Street, New York, NY 10014.

Publisher: *Marie Butler-Knight*
Editorial Director: *Mike Sanders*
Senior Managing Editor: *Billy Fields*
Acquisitions Editor: *Tom Stevens*
Senior Production Editor: *Megan Douglass*
Copy Editor: *Krista Hansing Editorial Services, Inc.*

Cartoonist: *Steve Barr*
Cover Designer: *Bill Thomas*
Book Designer: *Trina Wurst*
Indexer: *Tonya Heard*
Layout: *Ayanna Lacey*
Proofreader: *Mary Hunt*

Contents at a Glance

Contents

Appendixes

Introduction

Whether you're coping with a milk allergy, suffer from lactose intolerance, or are simply looking to cut back on milk and other dairy products, you've definitely come to the right place. Whatever your goals, let this book be your guide to the world of dairy-free eating.

We know that embarking on a new endeavor, particularly something like a dairy-free diet, can be a bit stressful and confusing at times, but we're here to provide you with the answers to your most pressing questions—before you even ask them! In the following chapters, you'll learn all about what's involved in taking the dairy-free plunge and how you can make your life and the lives of your family a lot easier—and delicious, of course—all without dairy.

After a few informative introductory chapters, we give you more than a dozen chapters chock full of wonderful dairy-free recipes, from breakfast to dessert, and everything in between. After trying some of these recipes, you'll be well on your way to becoming quite the dairy-free queen (or king). And don't be surprised if, when you head to the kitchen, you have quite a following—maybe even some folks who aren't dairy-conscious but can't wait to taste your next creation!

How This Book Is Organized

This book is divided into five parts:

Part 1, "The Dairy-Free Way," answers your questions about why and how to eliminate dairy from your diet. We also guide you on setting up your dairy-free kitchen and pantry, and introduce some of the remarkable ingredients you'll be getting to know.

Part 2, "Fresh Starts," is your guide to enjoying dairy-free breakfasts and brunches, with some terrific makeovers of dairy-rich dishes and suggestions for hot beverages and refreshing drinks.

Part 3, "Appetizers and Light Fare," provides you with tasty snacks, hors d'oeuvres, sandwiches, soups, and salads that fit the dairy-free bill without sacrificing flavor or creamy consistency.

Part 4, "What's for Dinner?" is your gateway to creating the most satisfying and tasty meals around, all without a drop of dairy. From beef entrées to poultry, pasta, vegetarian selections, and side dishes, you won't miss a thing when dairy is off the menu.

Part 5, "Amazing Desserts," proves that dairy free doesn't mean delicious free, with recipes for cookies, cakes, pudding, pies, and of course, dairy-free ice cream! You may be tempted to start right here after you see the array of possibilities.

Extras

Throughout the book, we've sprinkled boxed notes that offer you a little extra information. Here's what to look for:

 Dairy Don't _____
Be sure to heed these warnings and alerts about dairy-free matters.

 Milk-Free Morsel _____
These tips and hints are designed to make your dairy-free cooking and eating a bit easier.

 Lactose Lingo _____
Here you'll find helpful definitions of some unusual terms and ingredients.

 Free Fact _____
These boxes contain a wealth of facts and figures, as well as a little fun trivia.

Food Allergy Warning Icons

Because some food allergies can have dangerous consequences to some people, we've included warning icons to help easily identify whether a recipe contains ingredients like egg, gluten, soy, peanuts, tree nuts, fish, shellfish, and sesame:

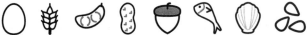

Acknowledgments

We would like to thank the staff at Alpha Books, particularly Tom Stevens and Christy Wagner, for their terrific support and patience. Marilyn Allen at the Allen O'Shea Literary Agency also deserves our gratitude. Thanks as well to Marion Groetch for her expertise, and everyone else who made this book possible and such a pleasure to create.

Special Thanks to the Technical Reviewer

The Complete Idiot's Guide to Dairy-Free Eating was reviewed by an expert who double-checked the accuracy of what you'll learn here, to help us ensure that this book gives you everything you need to know about feeding yourself and your family without the worry of hidden dairy products. Special thanks are extended to Jennifer S. Anderson.

Trademarks

All terms mentioned in this book that are known to be or are suspected of being trademarks or service marks have been appropriately capitalized. Alpha Books and Penguin Group (USA) Inc. cannot attest to the accuracy of this information. Use of a term in this book should not be regarded as affecting the validity of any trademark or service mark.

Part 1

The Dairy-Free Way

Part 1 explores what dairy-free eating really means, from the reasons to avoid dairy, to the ins and outs of eating dairy free on a daily basis. We look at what it means to have a milk allergy and how to best protect yourself from what could become severe allergic reactions. We also talk about lactose intolerance, a familiar problem for many but one not often fully understood. We show you how to identify hidden dairy in common foods and help you set up your kitchen for safe and delicious dairy-free cooking, including making your shopping list for excellent dairy product substitutes.

Armed with the information in Part 1, you'll be well prepared to plunge head first into dairy-free eating and cooking.

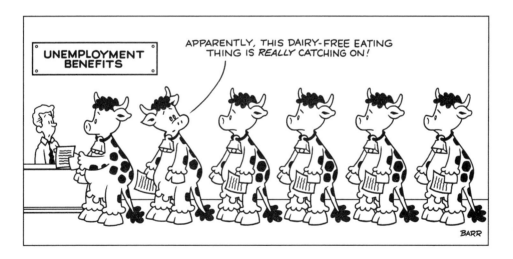

All About Dairy-Free Eating

In This Chapter

- Why go dairy free?
- Spotting dairy—even the hidden stuff
- Thriving with a dairy-free life

People choose to put milk out to pasture and avoid all milk and dairy products for all types of reasons, whether for personal convictions (such as vegans) or to follow a religious stricture (such as kosher). Others may have health concerns, such as milk allergies or lactose intolerance. For people with severe milk allergies, strictly avoiding even trace amounts of milk protein is required.

In this chapter, we take a close look at all things dairy and explore why dairy-free eating may be for you. In addition, we delve into the details of two particularly important reasons for going dairy free: milk allergy (an often serious and life-threatening issue) and lactose intolerance. You also learn why dairy can be taboo and how to avoid it day-to-day. By the end of this chapter, you'll have all the knowledge you need to avoid dairy in its many forms—in particular, places where dairy may unexpectedly lurk.

Milk: The Crème de la Crème?

Milk and dairy products are primarily derived from cow's milk, although the milk from other mammals such as sheep or goats may also be used in dairy-based items.

Cow's milk is perfectly formulated for complete nutrition for calves—baby cows, that is—just like human milk is perfectly formulated for human infants. But cow's milk is *not* appropriate for human babies, although a variety of infant formulas are derived from cow's milk. However, manufactured infant formulas make changes in the cow's milk to allow babies to drink it and stay healthy. If newborn babies were fed whole mammalian milks without these changes, they would become ill. (See Appendix C for more on infant formulas.)

What's Milk Got?

Whole cow's milk contains a variety of proteins, including the most abundant, *casein* and *whey* proteins. The proteins in milk account for one of the major problems associated with dairy: allergies. Milk also contains sugar, called lactose, which is a problem for people who are *lactose intolerant*, or have trouble digesting it. (More about lactose intolerance later in this chapter.)

> **Lactose Lingo**
>
> **Casein** and **whey** are two types of protein in cow's milk. Casein is found in all dairy products, including cheese, milk, and yogurt, and is often added to many processed foods. Whey is also found in all dairy products. It's abundant in the liquid that remains when casein is removed from milk, and is often dried and added to commercial foods and products.

Moo Juice Nutrients

Cow's milk also contains fats, the amount of which may vary depending on how the milk is processed. For example, whole milk is about 3.7 percent fat, whereas skim milk is about 0.5 percent milk fat and nonfat milk has no fat. Milk also has nutrients, including vitamins and minerals. In particular, milk is often fortified with vitamins A and D, and is a good source of calcium.

Because of these beneficial contents, whole cow's milk is considered a good source of nutrition for children. Adults, on the other hand, might prefer milks that are processed to reduce the fat and caloric content, to maintain or achieve a healthy weight. However, for all its healthy claims, the nutrients in cow's milk are not unique and can easily be obtained from other foods (as you'll see in Chapter 2).

All About Milk Allergy

It's important to distinguish between an allergy to milk and an intolerance. The differences are striking, and both the symptoms and treatment are diverse.

A *milk allergy* occurs when the immune system, the part of the body designed to fight infection, mistakenly attacks one or more of the proteins in milk. A variety of illnesses can result from this immune system attack, some of which can be severe and life-threatening.

A milk intolerance, also known as lactose intolerance, has nothing to do with the immune system: it refers to a lack of or reduced amount of an enzyme, called lactase, which is necessary for digesting milk. (You learn all about lactose intolerance later in this chapter.)

> **Lactose Lingo**
>
> A **milk allergy** is an immune system reaction to contact with milk proteins, resulting in sudden or chronic symptoms that may be life-threatening.

Antibodies on the Attack

When milk allergy is present, the immune system can attack in one of two main ways: one results in sudden symptoms and the other produces chronic symptoms.

In the first form of milk allergy, the immune system makes a protein called an IgE antibody that's able to recognize milk proteins. This antibody sits on the surface of the allergy cells throughout the body and acts like an antenna. When milk is ingested, the IgE antibody detects it and then signals the allergy cells to release a variety of chemicals, such as histamine, that cause symptoms of an allergic reaction. This type of allergic response typically comes on quickly, within minutes or an hour after the milk protein is ingested. It can result in skin rashes, sudden stomach problems, breathing trouble, and even problems with blood circulation.

> **Free Fact**
>
> Milk allergy is estimated to affect about 2.5 percent of young children. Although studies are limited, there is evidence suggesting that milk allergy prevalence has doubled in the past 3 decades.

Different from sudden allergic reactions but still troubling is when immune system cells in the body that are able to recognize milk proteins release chemicals that cause a variety of illnesses, usually affecting digestion or causing persistent itchy skin rashes. It's estimated that about half of young children with milk allergy have immediate reactions (and IgE antibodies to milk, to go along with it), while the remainder have more chronic types of milk allergic disease affecting the gut or skin. Interestingly, it's relatively rare for an adult to have or develop a life-threatening milk allergy.

Recognizing Allergic Symptoms

Although allergic reactions in general can be triggered by any number of sources, when the symptoms happen in relation to ingesting dairy, a milk allergy is something to consider. Symptoms of a milk allergy are divided between those that are sudden and those that are more chronic.

These sudden symptoms can occur together or separately:

◆ Skin rashes, itchiness, hives or welts, and swelling of the lips, eyelids, or face

◆ Itchy rashes

◆ Breathing problems, including wheezing, throat tightness or closing, inability to swallow, drooling, coughing, blue appearance, and a runny or blocked nose

◆ Stomach issues, including nausea, vomiting, diarrhea, and stomach pain or cramping

◆ Blood circulatory issues, such as paleness, confusion, fainting episodes, and loss of or weakness in pulse

◆ An itchy mouth

◆ A feeling of anxiety or doom

These chronic or daily ongoing symptoms can occur together or separately:

◆ Itchy skin rashes

◆ Stomach pain

◆ Vomiting

◆ Diarrhea

◆ Poor growth

Many reactions that could signal a milk allergy also could be caused by allergies to other types of food or could result from a variety of medical conditions that may have nothing to do with allergies. Always review your suspicions of milk, food, or other allergies with your doctor before making drastic dietary changes.

Diagnosing Milk Allergy

The most important test to diagnose a milk allergy is a patient's medical history. No laboratory tests can definitively diagnose a milk allergy—or an intolerance, for that matter—which is why a medical history is key. Any tests that are conducted are interpreted alongside the personal information you provide.

For example, your doctor will want to narrow the possibility of other foods and triggers that may be causing your symptoms by investigating their relationship to milk. Are the symptoms always related to milk consumption? How long after having milk do the symptoms start? Do symptoms depend on how much milk is consumed? It may be helpful to keep a diary of what you (or your child) eat and drink, along with any reactions related to those foods, beverages, or other products. The more information you can provide, the more likely you and your doctor will get to the root of the problem.

> **Free Fact**
>
> The good news about milk allergy is that those who suffer from it usually outgrow it. Most studies indicate an 85 percent or higher resolution rate by age 5. However, one recent study indicated that 20 percent were still allergic by their teen years.

Allergy skin tests, typically conducted by allergists, can detect the presence of IgE antibodies, often present in people who experience a sudden allergic reaction to dairy. In this simple test, an extract of milk is scratched into the skin using a small plastic probe or needle. If positive, the test results in a small itchy bump, like a mosquito bite.

Be aware, however, that this test, like many other tests conducted to determine the presence of disease, is not perfect. Having a positive allergy skin test to milk does not necessarily indicate a milk allergy. Some people may test positive but appear to handle dairy products just fine. On the other hand, it is possible to have problems with milk even though the test is negative, because the illness may be one not associated with IgE antibodies. Again, your medical history plays a huge role in interpreting any test results.

Allergy blood tests may also detect the presence of IgE antibodies to milk proteins. The rules for interpreting these tests are similar to the skin tests. A positive test may raise suspicion of a milk allergy but is not necessarily proof that one exists.

If chronic allergy symptoms could be related to dairy but the medical history and allergy tests do not give a clear diagnosis, your doctor may have you (or your child) undergo an elimination diet, a trial of avoiding dairy to see if any chronic symptoms go away.

The most definitive test to diagnose a milk allergy is a doctor-supervised gradual feeding of dairy called an oral food challenge. The doctor, usually an allergist, watches as dairy is gradually eaten, looking for any signs of a problem. This feeding test might be undertaken after a trial of dairy elimination or when the medical history and allergy tests do not otherwise confirm an allergy. Obviously, if there's a concern about severe reactions, like *anaphylaxis*, this feeding test is done with tiny amounts at a time in a setting where an allergic reaction can be treated.

> **Lactose Lingo**
>
> **Anaphylaxis** is a serious allergic reaction that comes on quickly after milk is ingested and could be fatal. Symptoms can include any of those occurring during a sudden allergic reaction, but the life-threatening symptoms of breathing difficulties and poor blood circulation are of highest concern.

Milk and Other Allergies

People with a cow's milk allergy are at increased risk for other allergies. Milk is on a rather short list of foods that account for most allergic reactions to food; others include eggs, peanuts, tree nuts, fish, shellfish, wheat, soy, and seeds.

> **Free Fact**
>
> Peanuts are technically not nuts, but legumes, and as such are not included in the usual allergy list of nuts or tree nuts. Interestingly, studies suggest that peanut allergy has doubled among children in the past decade.

In general, people with food allergies are commonly allergic to more than one type of food. Many young children with a milk allergy have additional food allergies, most often including one or more of the following: eggs, peanuts, wheat, soy, tree nuts, fish, and shellfish. It is possible, however, to have an allergy to *any* food, so always discuss these concerns with your doctor.

Treating Milk Allergy

The primary treatment of milk allergy is, quite simply, to avoid milk and all dairy products. However, that's easier said than done, and as vigilant as we may be, honest mistakes or unwanted surprises can occur. Being mindful of the following three basic rules for living with an allergy to milk will put you in good stead:

- Avoidance is key.

- Emergency plans should be in place.

- Education is essential.

Avoiding milk can be a very tricky prospect. Milk and other dairy products not only are everywhere in foods, but they also can lurk in some extremely unexpected places and circumstances. For example, a splash of milk in your kitchen could find its way into unintended foods, or butter could be added to a restaurant dish with very little thought. And remember, lactose-free milk and dairy products *are not safe* for people with milk allergy. Lactose free does not mean dairy free.

In addition, dairy can come in many different forms or can be hidden in some unlikely products you'd never think would contain dairy. Even a mother's breast milk can carry cow's milk proteins from her diet in small amounts, in which case Mom may need to eliminate or reduce the amount of milk she consumes while breast-feeding.

To increase your chances of successful avoidance, it's important to familiarize yourself with product labels—how to read them and what terms to look for. It also helps to be an active participant in situations where food is prepared and consumed, whether at school, in restaurants, at friends' homes, or in your own home. We look at this proactive stance in more detail later in this chapter; in the meantime, know that avoidance, whenever and wherever possible, is key.

Free Fact

Some children who are allergic to milk can tolerate small amounts of milk and other dairy products when the products are cooked or baked. It's believed that the high heat alters the milk protein enough to make it less problematic. Along the same lines, about 10 percent of children with severe milk allergy react to beef because it has some residual proteins found in both the milk and the meat. Sometimes cooking the beef longer reduces this allergy.

The primary treatment for a severe reaction to milk is a prompt injection of a prescription medication called epinephrine (adrenaline), available from your doctor as a self-injector. For those diagnosed with a severe or potentially severe milk allergy, the medication must be readily available in case of a severe allergic reaction.

Epinephrine reverses the severe symptoms of anaphylaxis, the breathing and blood circulation symptoms, giving time to get additional help, call 911, or get to an emergency room. Epinephrine works by opening clogged breathing tubes, reducing swelling, making the heart beat stronger, and making blood vessels carry blood more effectively—all good things to reverse the dangerous symptoms of anaphylaxis. Epinephrine's side effects include a racing heartbeat and jitteriness. They're generally short lived and not dangerous, compared to not treating anaphylaxis. Ask your doctor if you're concerned about side effects.

Self-injectors come in different strengths prescribed based on a child's weight; an adult dose is also available. Dummy injectors are available for practice. However, don't mix them up with the real ones. Always read manufacturer inserts for instructions and care, and check the label for expiration dates.

An injection should certainly be administered if milk was accidentally ingested and symptoms of breathing troubles or poor circulation develop. (See "Recognizing Allergic Symptoms," earlier in this chapter.) However, you can give epinephrine during an allergic reaction before severe symptoms develop. For example, if you notice the progression of hives, swelling, and/or vomiting, it's best to inject. Similarly, if there's a history of a very severe allergic reaction, you may want to inject the epinephrine if you know milk was ingested, even before any significant symptoms start. When in doubt, it's generally better to inject. Just remember the old adage to "shoot first and ask questions later." (Your doctor can tell you more about this.) Finally, sometimes a second dose of epinephrine is needed if symptoms are not improving or if they come back after a first dose before receiving medical attention. Because of this possibility, doctors typically prescribe two doses to be carried at all times.

> ⊘ **Dairy Don't** _____
>
> Anaphylaxis can be fatal. You must receive medical attention for anaphylaxis, even if symptoms improve after the epinephrine. Because reactions may return, staying under supervision in an emergency room for at least 4 hours is imperative.

Asthma treatments such as inhaled bronchodilators that open clogged breathing tubes may reduce wheezing during anaphylaxis, but they _should not be expected or depended on to treat anaphylaxis_. Antihistamines help to reduce itch and swelling and are good treatments for an allergic reaction or anaphylaxis, but they also _cannot replace_ *epinephrine* to treat anaphylaxis. Work with your doctor to learn how and when to use the epinephrine self-injector so you are always prepared. A written emergency plan, created with your doctor, is highly recommended.

Whenever you're dealing with a chronic disease or illness, educating yourself on the subject can often be your best ammunition. But educating others in your circle of activities can be dramatically beneficial as well. Anyone who comes in contact with someone coping with milk allergy—teachers, school nurses, parents of children's friends, or camp counselors—should be alerted to the allergy and provided the emergency plan. It's also helpful to purchase medical identification jewelry so everyone within and without your immediate circle can be easily alerted, too.

> **Free Fact**
>
> Children who have milk or other food allergies are at higher risk to develop respiratory allergies triggered by dust, pollen, and animal dander, to name a few, manifesting as asthma and hay fever, also called allergic rhinitis. The progression of allergy problems from food allergy to respiratory allergies is called the allergic march.

All About Lactose Intolerance

Lactose is the name of the sugar in mammalian milk. *Lactase* is an enzyme that breaks down that milk sugar. When lactase "digests" lactose, smaller sugars of lactose are absorbed as nutrients. If there's a deficiency of lactase, meaning less of the enzyme, the lactose passes along the intestine undigested and unabsorbed, causing trouble in a variety of ways. Gut bacteria can get hold of the lactose and ferment it, causing gas, and the extra sugar in the intestine can draw fluids out of the body and into the gut, causing diarrhea. All this is called *lactose intolerance*. An estimated 70 percent of the world's population has a poor ability to digest milk sugar. That means it is normal to be lactose intolerant, at least as an adult.

> **Lactose Lingo**
>
> **Lactose** is the sugar present in milk. **Lactase** is the enzyme required to digest lactose. An inability to properly digest lactose is called **lactose intolerance.**

Babies need to be able to digest the milk sugar in their mother's milk, so babies have enough lactase to do the job. But nature probably didn't expect people to continue to consume mother's milk past the first year or 2 of life, and after that time, the levels of gut lactase enzymes gradually decline. There are racial and ethnic differences in the loss of lactase into adulthood. Persons of Asian descent have the highest rates of lactase deficiency, at more than 90 percent. More than 70 percent of Native Americans and African Americans have lactase deficiency, and the lowest rates, 5 to 20 percent, are among Caucasian adults. The rate at which lactase levels decrease over time as a person ages is also racially and ethnically related. For example, Chinese and Japanese lose 80 to 90 percent within a few years after breast-feeding, Jews and Asians 60 to 70 percent, while white Northern Europeans may reach their lowest level of lactase after the age of 20.

Other instances can lead to lactose intolerance as well. Having a stomach virus can result in temporary loss of lactase for days or weeks. And some infants have a rare medical condition in which they are born without lactase and suffer from lactose intolerance throughout life. Similarly rare is a medical disorder known as Galactosemia that can occur when the sugar galactose, created by the digestion of lactose, can cause severe damage to the liver, kidney, brain, and eyes. For the most part, however, lactose intolerance is a normal part of human aging.

Signs of Trouble

Symptoms of lactose intolerance include diarrhea, cramps, bloating, flatulence, and, less commonly, nausea and vomiting after eating dairy. Typically, these symptoms develop between 30 minutes and several hours after consumption of dairy.

Lactose intolerance can be characterized in two ways: one is by the severity of the symptoms, and the other is by the amount of lactose that triggers a reaction. This variability may be due to the amount of enzyme a person has and the amount and types of natural bacteria in the gut that also digest lactose, among other individual reasons. Some people are very sensitive, so a very small amount of lactose bothers them; others can tolerate rather large amounts—even cups of milk—before having symptoms.

Diagnosing Your Condition

Unlike the methods and tests used to diagnose milk allergy, generally all that's needed to determine lactose intolerance is realizing a connection between your symptoms and the fact that you've eaten dairy products. Avoiding lactose for a few days and watching for a resolution of symptoms—while also noting the recurrence of symptoms after lactose is added back—is the usual method of diagnosis; in most cases, individuals can do this without a physician's assistance. For example, it may be helpful to do a trial in a very regimented way by keeping a symptom diary for several days before going off lactose-containing foods, and then noting your reactions for several days in a row while free of lactose. End your test with several days back on lactose, and compare your symptoms, watching for important connections.

In addition to self-testing, a breath hydrogen test can diagnose lactose intolerance. Under a doctor's assessment, a lactose-containing liquid is taken. Several hours later, the individual gives a breath sample that's measured for hydrogen content: the hydrogen level is elevated if the lactose is not being absorbed. The test is not foolproof, however, and may miss the diagnosis up to 20 percent of the time.

Free Fact

Irritable bowel syndrome (IBS) includes symptoms of abdominal pain, bloating, diarrhea, and constipation and, therefore, shares symptoms with lactose intolerance. Some people have both lactose intolerance and IBS. Eliminating dairy may improve IBS, whether or not lactose intolerance is also present.

Treating Lactose Intolerance

Unlike people with severe milk allergy, people with lactase deficiency can usually tolerate small or even modest amounts of dairy, especially as part of a meal, as opposed to drinking a glass of milk on its own. Symptoms can usually be avoided by spreading out the consumption of lactose-rich products over the course of a day and eating or drinking less at a specific meal.

If you are lactose intolerant, you might try commercially available dairy products that are "predigested," or processed with enzymes. These are labeled *lactose free* and may help some people avoid the symptoms of lactose intolerance. When a lactose-rich meal cannot be avoided, supplemental lactase enzymes, or lactase pills, may be helpful as well. These are taken in either chewable or dissolvable form at the first bite of a meal or drink containing dairy, and are generally safe to use.

Contrary to common belief, fermented milk products, including cheese and yogurt, often do not lead to symptoms of lactose intolerance because lactic acid bacteria

Free Fact

Some pill or capsule forms of medications can have lactose as a filler, although the amount is extremely small and usually tolerated.

in the foods help digest the lactose. In addition, some cheeses, such as camembert, cheddar, cream cheese, and Parmesan, contain less lactose and may not induce a reaction. However, most dairy products normally contain about 4 or 5 percent lactose by weight—enough to create symptoms in lactose-intolerant people.

Defining Dairy Products

You only need to stroll down the dairy aisle of your supermarket to find the dairy products, right? Well, not exactly. You will find many dairy products there, but many other supermarket aisles contain milk products and other dairy items as well. The only way to truly know whether a product you're buying contains dairy is to read the label—and sometimes even that proves a bit challenging.

Interpreting Product Labels

The Food Allergen Labeling and Consumer Protection Act requires that foods with milk ingredients use the term *milk* on the label either in the ingredient list or in a separate *Contains milk* statement. A label can use scientific words for milk proteins, such as *casein* or *whey*, but the word *milk* must also appear on the label. The following buzz words may indicate milk ingredients, too: *artificial butter flavor, butter fat, butter, butter oil, casein/caseinates, cream, curd, custard, ghee, lactalbumin, lactoglobulin, lactoferrin, lactulose, nougat, pudding, rennet, Recaldent* (used in certain teeth-whitening products and gums), *Simpless, whey, yogurt.*

Labeling laws do not currently regulate allergen advisory warnings such as *may contain milk, processed on equipment that processes milk,* or *made in a facility that processes milk.* A manufacturer puts these warnings on its products at its own discretion and uses words it deems appropriate. The Food and Drug Administration simply requires that such labeling be truthful.

Foods marked *nondairy* can often contain milk proteins. Marketed to primarily lactose-intolerant consumers, nondairy products simply mean they're not primarily milk based compared to their dairy-containing counterparts. *Dairy-free* labeling, however, means what it says.

Free Fact

Based on studies done with peanut allergen advisory labels, it's believed that risk-related words on product labels can't be trusted to be accurate. For example, *produced in a facility with milk* is not necessarily lower risk than *may contain milk.*

Read the ingredient label every time you purchase a product, and look over the entire label, including under any folds or flaps. Even though you may have safely examined the label in the past, read it each time you purchase the product because. manufacturers often change ingredients for any number of reasons.

Moreover, be aware that nutritional supplements and vitamins may contain milk but are not covered by labeling laws. Neither are cosmetics, shampoos, and medications. In some cases, contacting the manufacturer may be the only way to determine whether a product is dairy free.

Is That Kosher?

Many people eat a kosher diet. In essence, it is forbidden to consume dairy with meat, so religious food labeling has added the easily recognized term *pareve* to indicate that a product does not contain milk. However, the *pareve* label can be ambiguous, and we mustn't put total faith in the claim: small amounts of milk protein may actually be present in these products and still be designated as pareve. As small as these amounts may be, they may still be enough to trigger an allergic reaction in those who have milk allergy, so be mindful of this type of labeling and don't take chances.

As a help to consumers, most products now display kosher dairy symbols, such as a *D* next to a circled *k* or *U*, meaning the product has milk proteins.

Dairy and the Vegan Lifestyle

Unlike vegetarian eaters, who may choose to consume some types of dairy products, vegans neither use nor consume animal products, including dairy-containing products. For the most part, products safe for vegans are also safe for dairy-free eaters.

Manufacturers of vegan products can apply for certification so a *certified vegan* logo appears on their packaging. Although the ingredients of the products are certified to be animal free and, therefore, dairy free, the possibility of cross-contamination from machinery used for dairy and dairy-free items still may exist because this claim, when it appears, is only self-reported. To clear up any concerns, contact the manufacturer.

Counting Sheep (and Goats)

Most people with a cow's milk allergy are also allergic to milk from sheep, ewe, goats, and buffalo. This phenomenon, known as *cross-reactivity*, can result in the same allergic symptoms experienced with cow-based dairy products.

> **Lactose Lingo** _____
>
> **Cross-reactivity** means that an allergy to one food substance may result in an allergy to another food that has similar proteins.

Many cheeses, such as chevre (goat), some types of mozzarella (buffalo), and feta (sheep), fall into this category, and it isn't unusual these days to find quarts of goat's milk right alongside quarts of cow's milk or soy milk in the supermarket. Sometimes it's possible to be allergic to the milk derived from these other animals and not be allergic to cow's milk. Your doctor can help you determine whether this might be the case.

Animals whose milk appears much less likely to induce allergic reactions among people with cow's milk allergy are camels, mules, and donkeys, although rarely are these animals used as a milk source.

Avoiding Dairy Away from Home

In Chapter 2, you learn everything you need to know to keep a dairy-free kitchen, but what about when you're away from the safety of home? Is it possible to have any control over what you're fed as you venture out into the world? Keep reading for the tips and advice you need to maintain a dairy-free diet when eating out.

Check, Please ... and Please Check!

Eating out should be a treat for the whole family. But when concerns about milk allergy and intolerance are front and center in your mind, how can you enjoy the experience without trepidation? Learning a little bit about how restaurant kitchens are run and not being afraid to ask for special attention are two ways to ensure your dining experience is a pleasant one and not a cause for anxiety or panic.

Most higher-end restaurant menus include the ingredients contained in special dishes with enticing descriptions. However, this doesn't mean the ingredient list is complete. The only way to truly know whether what you're ordering contains dairy is to ask the cook or chef. Even the server may not have all the answers, so don't be afraid to go to the source. Most fine dining chefs know their ingredients well and can tell you whether a dish contains milk, butter, or cheese, at the very least. They can also tell you if they're able to make a dish dairy free for you as a special request. Traces of milk protein as a hidden ingredient, however, is another story, and this is where you need to be proactive, particularly if milk allergy is your concern.

Consider creating a "Chef Card" that lists your milk allergy and any other food allergies you may have, as well as any unexpected dairy-containing ingredients you avoid and common pitfalls that might occur in the kitchen. You can find an example at www.foodallergy.org to follow as a guide. To be fair, always emphasize to the staff that this is an allergy issue and a critical health concern, not simply a personal preference or dictation of how they should do their job. Most people are more than happy to oblige if possible when approached with courtesy and understanding.

In more casual dining establishments, menus are often created by franchises or head cooks who may not even be on the premises at all times. Many meals may even include some prepackaged or premade components, to ensure consistency in preparation. In these instances, it would be virtually impossible to make many special requests, so order something you know is safe. If you have any doubts, or if you're unable to get a definitive answer from the staff, choose something else. And always be sure to carry medication with you as your emergency plan.

 Dairy Don't

Cross-contact or cross-contamination can be a real concern. Dairy-free ingredients or meals that come in contact with dairy ingredients either by spillage or through shared utensils and equipment are no longer dairy free and can contain milk proteins by transference. Buffets and salad bars are notorious for this.

Back to School

Sending a child with milk allergy off to school or daycare can produce anxiety in a parent. If your child has a milk allergy, it's important to meet with school staff, including the school nurse, principal, food service manager, and teachers, early on to let them know a milk allergy exists. Your child's age is an important factor in deciding how best to keep him safe: younger and more impulsive children are more prone to take foods from others.

In a daycare setting, unfortunately, cross-contact can occur in numerous ways. Children could suck on toys, which might cause a reaction if another child had been drinking milk and left milk saliva on the toy. Messy cheesy snacks like puffed snacks and cheesy chips can spread dairy dust. Alternative snacks and hand washing may reduce the risks, but as always, communicating with the people in charge is your primary defense.

No matter what the age or school situation, be sure to meet with the staff before the school year starts and provide them with written documentation about the allergy. Include a written emergency treatment plan from your child's doctor that outlines the symptoms to look for, what treatments to give, and important contact information. Attach a picture of the child to the treatment plan, and provide labeled medications. Review how to avoid an allergic reaction and what will be done in the event of accidental ingestion. Finally, review with your child his own responsibilities for staying safe, such as not sharing or trading food, alerting an adult to symptoms, and if age appropriate, carrying and using his medication.

Free Fact _____

Severe reactions to milk occur primarily through ingestion. However, skin contact with milk can also trigger a reaction, most often leading to skin rashes or hives. Reactions from airborne contact is also a possibility if you're around steaming or boiling milk.

On the Road

As you travel on vacation, visit relatives and friends, or travel for sports activities or other functions, preparation can make all the difference. Being on the road means being away from the security and familiarity of home, but it doesn't have to be an uncomfortable experience if you do a little detective work ahead of time and have a good plan in place.

Free Fact _____

Currently, there's no cure for a milk allergy, and avoidance is the main treatment. However, a number of studies are showing that better treatments may be possible someday, by either blocking the allergic reactions or re-educating the immune system to stop attacking milk proteins.

To help you on the road, always carry your emergency medications, up-to-date and pharmacy labeled, with extras if you're traveling to remote or far locations. Call ahead to be sure safe foods are available, carry a backup food pack for unexpected situations, and consider booking a room with a kitchenette. Know where emergency health care is available at your destination and along the way, and carry your insurance and health information at all times. For air and foreign travel, have a doctor's note explaining the allergy and any need to carry foods or medications.

When visiting relatives or friends, or attending parties, it may be a good idea to bring much of your own food, to avoid problems and alleviate stress for your host. For a child going to a birthday party, consider calling ahead to find out what others will be eating, which may allow you to develop a similar dairy-free treat so your child doesn't feel left out.

Above all, remember to relax and have fun. Avoiding dairy should never mean avoiding life.

The Least You Need to Know

- A diet free of dairy may be desirable for a number of reasons, including milk allergy, lactose intolerance, or personal preference..

- Milk allergy, most prevalent in children, requires strict avoidance of dairy products and can result in severe reactions.

- Lactose intolerance, most prevalent in adults, is a normal condition that can improve through a dairy-free diet.

- Eating dairy free can be a challenge but is an attainable goal when preparation, education, and satisfying alternatives are provided.

Chapter 2

The Dairy-Free Kitchen

In This Chapter

- ◆ Gearing up to cook dairy free
- ◆ Discovering new ingredients and methods
- ◆ Advice on nutrition for dairy-free eaters

It's time to learn about the joys and, yes, the challenges of dairy-free cooking. Whether you're new to the kitchen or an old pro, you'll want to review the tips and information in this chapter so your quest for delicious dairy-free eating and cooking yields only delicious—and safe—results.

Giving Your Kitchen a Dairy-Free Makeover

Maintaining a dairy-free kitchen for those dealing with milk allergy, particularly a severe allergy, demands a clean and uncluttered work area and an organized pantry and fridge—even more so than the average household because of the danger of cross-contact with milk. For instance, maybe only one person in your family must avoid dairy, while others can quite happily indulge. Because you'll probably be buying and storing both dairy-free and dairy-containing products, it's important to keep the milk and milk products separate from the dairy-free items. Whether you appoint specific shelves and drawers for these items or simply remind family members of the danger of closeness, it's a concept everyone must bear in mind at all times.

> **Milk-Free Morsel**
>
> Wrapping foods securely with foil or plastic wrap and using airtight containers when appropriate to store dairy-free foods helps prevent cross-contact with milk products.

For those who aren't coping with milk allergy, the rules are certainly less stringent, but why not let organization be your motto anyway? Having an orderly kitchen where you can put your hands on exactly what you need without frantically scouring drawers and shelves, tossing items here and there like a cat burglar searching for the family jewels, is practically every home cook's dream. Here's your excuse to put everything in its place.

Clear Out the Cupboards

Sifting through your cupboard and pantry ingredients, regardless of specific dietary requirements, is something everyone should do on a regular basis. This way, you can eliminate expired items, flours and grains that might have become "buggy" (don't deny you've seen that—we all have), or stale products that were harmed by temperature extremes or improper repackaging.

After you've sorted everything and separated the "keepers" from the "has-beens," give your cupboard and/or pantry shelves a good cleaning with hot, soapy water. Dry well and, if they don't have them already, consider applying shelf liners to the clean surfaces.

Now it's time to do a little label reading to unearth some hidden dairy ingredients. Look for the buzz words listed in Chapter 1 and, if in doubt, toss it or put it aside. Labels with *casein*, *whey*, and, of course, *milk* are obvious, but be sure to examine all those impossible-to-pronounce ingredients as well.

> **Dairy Don't**
>
> Believe it or not, some household products such as shampoos, lotions, and even pet food can contain milk proteins. As always, read your labels!

When you're satisfied with your detective work, wipe clean the containers or boxes and put them back on the clean shelf in an orderly, organized manner. You can write on the shelf paper with a felt-tip marker to quickly describe the types of ingredients one will find there. For example, "Dairy-free," "No milk," or even something like "Emily's shelf" will get the message across to everyone.

Cool Storage Care

Just as you did with your pantry items, you'll want to remove everything from the fridge and check for expiration dates and any deterioration in quality. When everything's out, a serious cleaning with hot, soapy water is in order—include drawers and shelves. Once again, check products for dairy buzz words and return them, containers wiped clean, to the fridge. If you're designating shelves for dairy-free items, you can adhere some electrical tape to the plastic or glass and write on it with a permanent marker. Keeping dairy-free milks and products on the uppermost shelves helps prohibit unwanted drips and splashes from regular cow's milk and related items.

Don't forget your freezer in your kitchen makeover. You'll need a designated area there as well to make room for all those delicious dairy-free ice creams you'll be making!

Clean = Safe

Don't ignore counters, stovetops, tables, and any other surfaces in the kitchen that have been yearning for a good scrub. You'll need to clean these areas on a regular basis, so you might as well begin the habit now. In addition, cutting boards should be well cleaned, and you may even want to consider purchasing separate cutting boards for dairy and nondairy.

> **Milk-Free Morsel**
>
> Consider preparing the dairy-free meal before the regular meal, to reduce the risk of cross-contact. Pans or grills used to make cheeseburgers, for instance, could contaminate a cheese-free burger, and utensils used to sauté vegetables that have butter added could end up transferring milk protein to dairy-free vegetables.

There! That wasn't so bad, was it? Now you're ready to meet your new dairy-free ingredients that will be helping you discover how delicious and rewarding dairy-free eating and cooking can be.

How Now, Brown Cow?

Is it really possible to enjoy food without sweet cream, rich butter, or a tall, cold glass of milk? You bet! Today we are afforded a good selection of basic dairy-free products that were unheard of years ago. Back when soy milk was available only in cartons at room temperature and fake cheese had the flavor of soapsuds, dairy-free eaters were pretty much limited in the shopping department—even then, it had to be at the local health food store where the "hippies" shopped.

Now we see refrigerated soy milk—in several different flavors—alongside cow's milk in the "dairy" section. Your local supermarket may even have a whole area of organic, vegan, and dairy-free products where you can choose everything from chocolate almond milk to vegan Parmesan cheese. If you've never explored these areas, you're in for a real treat.

The Wonderful World of Soy

If it's been a long time since you've tried soy milk and other soy products, assuming no allergy issues are at stake, it's time you reintroduced yourself to all soy has to offer. The variety and quality available will really surprise you, and in many cases, you'll be able to substitute soy milk and its related soy-based food items on a one-to-one basis for recipes that call for milk and milk products. From sour cream to cream cheese to yogurt, you'll pretty much find a soy substitute to fit the bill. Beware, however, that some soy products can contain milk protein, so always read labels before you buy.

Next to sushi, Japan's gift to the culinary world most certainly is tofu. These days tofu appears in almost every supermarket, as well as on many restaurant menus. The great thing about tofu is that it has the ability to absorb any flavors you want to impart. As a result, it can compliment a dish without interfering with its ultimate taste. A great source of protein, tofu has been turned into everything from "ice cream" to "chicken nuggets."

Soy milk, soy products, and tofu are only the opening act for dairy-free eating and cooking, and you'll want to check out many more remarkable dairy-free products. Come on, we'll introduce you.

More Milk, Please

Almond milk is destined to become one of your favorite new friends. Made from ground almonds and filtered water, it has a light consistency and a delicate almond flavor, often perfect for beverage and dessert concoctions. Available plain or unsweetened, as well as in vanilla and chocolate flavors, you'll find a variety of places for almond milk in your dairy-free kitchen. Savory dishes can benefit from a bit of almond milk creaminess when flavor appropriate, so don't assume it's only for drinking or baking. You can find almond milk in aseptic cartons at room temperature. After you open it, store it in the refrigerator, where it will keep for 7 to 10 days.

Rice milk will also pleasantly surprise you. Sometimes found refrigerated in the dairy section, rice milk can add just the right amount of faux milk without interfering with flavor like soy or almond milk sometimes does. Typically made from brown rice and filtered water, it has a bit of natural sweetness all its own and is often available without any added sugar. Some people actually prefer rice milk to other milk substitutes because of its subtle flavor, and it's a real life saver for those coping with soy and tree nut allergies, as well as an allergy to cow's milk. Available in many flavors, rice milk generally keeps refrigerated for up to 10 days.

Other types of milk you may find in your dairy-free hunt are oat milk, whole-grain milk, and even potato milk. If you're feeling adventurous, try some of these more unusual products—you might just hit on a new favorite.

One of the beneficial aspects of commercially produced milk substitutes is that they're usually fortified with vitamins and minerals, particularly those that might be in short supply for dairy-free eaters. We discuss nutritional issues later in this chapter, but depending on your doctor's recommendations, you may want to purchase enhanced milk substitutes.

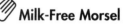 **Milk-Free Morsel**

If you're truly adventurous, you can try making milk substitute at home, including almond milk and rice milk. After soaking, refrigerating, and straining the source ingredient, you're left with the "milk." Various methods and techniques for milking are available online, so if the urge strikes you, definitely make an attempt.

Last but definitely not least is the wonderful product coconut milk. (In 2006, the Food and Drug Administration classified coconut as a tree nut, and although it had rarely been shunned by those with a tree nut allergy in the past, some doctors may advise against it. Check with yours to be sure.) Although coconut milk has a definite sweetness and distinct flavor, it has become a kitchen staple for many home cooks, particularly those who frequently prepare Asian cuisine. But don't stop there. Hot beverages, enticing desserts, and incomparable entrées of all types can benefit from coconut milk. Available canned, usually regular or light, and sweetened or unsweetened, it has a long shelf life unopened but needs to be kept in the refrigerator after it's opened. It will last there for about a week.

Cream of coconut, made from the coconut meat and cane sugar, is also an option in the dairy-free kitchen. However, be careful of grabbing "cream of coconut" or "coconut cream" products like mixers used in cocktail making because they may contain milk in some form. As always, label reading is a must.

Meet Your New Dairy-Free Staples

As we start to explore the concept of dairy-free cooking, it's often helpful to know what role dairy usually plays in a recipe, particularly before we decide on a specific substitute. For example, although it's clear that butter contributes richness and flavor wherever it appears, it may also be acting as a binder of sorts to keep the other ingredients in sauces, piecrusts, and cookies neatly together. Can this be accomplished by something else? Often the answer is yes. Healthy oils, from canola to olive, might happily step in as a substitute for butter. If flavor is the primary goal, then a dairy-free margarine that boasts "buttery taste" might be the preferred understudy. Or if creaminess is the desired result, a splash of soy creamer or coconut milk might be the answer.

For the majority of recipes out there, a simple substitute exists to make it dairy free. Let's take a closer look at some of the new dairy-free ingredients you'll be adding to your cast of characters in your new dairy-free kitchen.

Dairy-Free Margarine and Shortening

If you're alarmed by the idea of using margarine on a regular basis because of hydrogenation, it's time to take a close look at margarine. Since it was established that trans fats are undesirable, many margarine manufacturers have revamped their products to exclude it. Sure, some companies still use it, but for the most part, many more products are now nonhydrogenated and trans fat free. In most cases, the flavor of margarines has been vastly improved as well.

Whether you use tubs or sticks, dairy-free margarine will become a staple for many different types of recipes. Just be sure you read the label carefully: milk derivatives may find their way into the ingredient list.

Vegetable shortening may also become an ally, although most people have shunned its use for quite some time, again because of hydrogenation. But if soy is a problem for you, vegetable shortening may be the solution, because most margarines contain some amount of soy.

Healthful Oils

Oils made from vegetables, fruits, nuts, and seeds can add distinct flavor to a dish, as well as provide richness, binding ability, and texture. A moist carrot cake nearly always gets its consistency from vegetable oil (and carrots, of course), and is a recipe that is naturally dairy free (apart from the cream cheese frosting!).

Whether it's the fruitiness of an extra-virgin olive oil, the nuttiness of sesame oil, or the subtleness of canola oil, there's a place in the dairy-free kitchen for all of these oils when the occasion arises. Traditional butter sautéing can become delicious oil sautéing with the right choice, so be sure to keep a good supply of varied oils on hand.

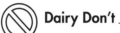 **Dairy Don't**

Some oils, particularly from nuts and seeds, need to be refrigerated because they can go rancid quite quickly at room temperature.

Creamers and Creams

Soy creamer will no doubt become one of your favorite ingredients. Available in the dairy section, it usually comes in both plain and vanilla flavors. With a consistency like half-and-half, soy creamer is perfect for adding to beverages, soups, sauces, and a variety of desserts, as well being a terrific ingredient for nondairy ice creams.

Be aware, however, that those nondairy creamers you may see alongside it are not necessarily dairy free. Unless they're specifically labeled *vegan*, they can potentially contain small amounts of milk protein.

Soy-based sour cream is a surprisingly good product and can be used in place of cow's milk sour cream. And dairy-free cream cheese, made from tofu, is terrific for filling the shoes of regular cream cheese, even as a replacement in that cream cheese frosting you'll want to make for your carrot cake! Soy yogurt is another winner and does quite well in blended drinks and desserts, whether flavored or plain. Do read labels, however, as small amounts of dairy can creep into some soy yogurts. Happily, the protein and healthy bacteria found in regular yogurt are also present in soy yogurt, so its content as well as its consistency make it a good team player.

Cheese Alternatives

Giving up cheese can be one of the more disappointing prospects of dairy-free eating, but thankfully, more good-quality faux cheese products are becoming available. Most are soy based, but look for the vegan certification to be sure no traces of milk are lurking.

Many of the new vegan cheeses are actually able to melt when heated, replicating that ooey-gooey consistency most people love. You can find a range of kinds to experiment with, from cheddars, to mozzarellas, to provolones, to Parmesans, to good old American-style offerings. Many faux cheeses come shredded as well as sliced. Do watch for the inclusion of nuts, however, if this is an issue; many cheese products incorporate them into their ingredients.

An unusual player for cheese substitution is nutritional yeast. Oddly enough, it has quite a cheesy flavor when added to dishes and does a terrific job creating sauces and the classic favorite macaroni and cheese.

Don't hesitate to give these products a try. They are often unexpectedly good.

Chocolate!

It's true! You don't have to give up chocolate! Apart from milk chocolate, darker chocolates with at least 50 percent cocoa content are, in most cases, safe for dairy-free eaters. Do read labels, however, just in case some type of milk protein is present. The higher the cocoa content, the less likely you will find any milk derivatives. There is the potential for cross contamination however, if a facility processes both milk and dark chocolate. If in doubt, look for certified vegan dark chocolate, which is dairy-free by definition.

White chocolate—which is really not chocolate at all, in the true sense—can often be found dairy free but, unfortunately, may contain hydrogenated oils. Moderate use may be the best approach. By the way, white chocolate's main ingredient, cocoa butter, does not contain dairy, in spite of its name. Similarly, chocolate liquor, which is present in milk and dark chocolate but absent from white chocolate, is not alcohol based—another misnomer.

Cocoa powder is also on any list of dairy-free staples, and if you don't have much experience with it, you'll be amazed at its intensity of flavor in baking.

> **Milk-Free Morsel**
>
> Don't be misled by misnomers. Cocoa butter, coconut butter, peanut butter, tree and seed butters, fruit butter, and butternut squash are all dairy free!

Eggs

A quick word about eggs: substituting for eggs in recipes may be necessary or desirable. In fact, a common allergy that accompanies milk allergy is an egg allergy, requiring double vigilance. Powdered egg replacer, prepared according to the package directions, can fill in nicely in these instances.

For those who can tolerate egg but prefer to use something lower in cholesterol and fat, refrigerated dairy-free egg substitutes are a fine alternative. Silken tofu, puréed pumpkin or banana, or applesauce ($1/4$ cup = 1 egg) can also be used in baking recipes.

Churning Up Consistency and Flavor

Making one-on-one dairy-free substitutions in recipes that call for milk and milk products is only one way to replace consistency and flavor. Chefs have a number of tricks up their sleeve to create just about any desired outcome, whether it be smooth and creamy, rich and buttery, or silky and sweet, and most rely on both technique and some unusual ingredients. Something "creamy" may actually have nothing to do with cream at all. How do they do it?

Mother Nature has supplied us with an abundant array of natural ingredients whose innate qualities often mimic textures and flavors of other foods:

◆ Yukon Gold potatoes are famous for their buttery taste and can contribute great flavor to recipes where butter might normally be found.

◆ Rice, when added to soups and blended with other ingredients, can result in a particularly creamy consistency without the use of cream or milk.

◆ Vegetables such as sweet potatoes and butternut squash, especially when roasted in the oven and allowed to caramelize, can be almost as sugary-sweet as candy.

◆ Rich and creamy beans of all sorts can mimic both cream and buttery thickeners, also called *roux*, when allowed to break down in stews and soups to thicken the consistency and flavor the outcome.

A number of easy-to-employ techniques result in a dish that would normally require dairy in some form to create texture, bind ingredients, or thicken resulting sauces or gravies. Making roux with oil instead of butter is an old Southern standard for gumbos and creoles, and along with its quintessential ingredient—okra—provides all that's needed for a thick and rich result.

Emulsification, which is simply the coming together of two ingredients such as oil and vinegar that normally do not combine well, can be accomplished through vigorous whisking or blending, to result in a silky consistency.

And adding ingredients like cornstarch or flour can make for creamy consistencies without the need for cream.

Meeting Nutritional Guidelines

As soon as you announce you're following a dairy-free diet, you'll probably encounter people who, for whatever reason, become immediately alarmed: *What about calcium? Aren't you afraid of osteoporosis? Isn't your child being deprived of important nutrition?*

Simply put, we have become convinced that life without milk is unhealthy, when in fact, nothing could be further from the truth.

More Than a Quest for Calcium

As you saw in Chapter 1, milk and milk products provide protein, fat, carbohydrates, and a multitude of vitamins and minerals, not least of which is calcium. Guess what? So do baked beans, although the fat content is nearly nonexistent, which isn't necessarily a bad thing.

So many other food items can provide the same nutrition you receive from cow's milk. The majority of milk's nutritional contents—protein; calcium; magnesium; vitamins C, D, A, K; and a number of B vitamins as well—are found in numerous food sources, including animal protein, fish, vegetables, grains, beans, nuts, and seeds.

Interestingly, when we examine and compare the absorption rate of, for example, the calcium found in milk (about 32 percent) to, say, kale (nearly 70 percent), where's the advantage? What's important to our bodies is the accessibility to nutrients present in the food we eat and the ease with which they can be assimilated. In other words, if we can't get to the calcium and absorb it, what does it matter that something has loads of calcium?

Supplemental Facts

Getting your calcium is more about absorbing it than ingesting it, and there are numerous reasons why, in addition to its accessibility in food, our ability may be compromised. Excess salt intake, smoking, alcohol abuse, caffeine, and lack of exercise can all contribute to a shortage of calcium in our bones.

Although nearly all women are encouraged to take calcium supplements, particularly after menopause, the ideal amount is still unclear. What appears to be more important, especially for women, is preventing the loss of calcium through lifestyle changes and sometimes medication.

In general, a well-balanced diet shouldn't necessarily require supplementation, but follow your doctor's lead on this, especially if you or someone in your family is embarking on a dairy-free diet. Children with milk allergy should be especially monitored for nutritional intake by a doctor and dietitian.

> **Free Fact**
>
> Yale University reviewed a number of international studies on women, osteoporosis, and dairy intake, and concluded that the countries with the highest rates of osteoporosis were also the highest consumers of dairy products.

Top Food Choices for Dairy-Free Eaters

Many of the dairy-free foods you'll be enjoying when you kick dairy to the curb are often fortified with calcium as well as other nutrients. But if you prefer to get your calcium directly from the source or are interested in eating foods with more bang for your buck, here's a list of calcium-rich dairy-free foods:

Acorn squash	Kiwi
Almonds	Papaya
Beans (white, black, baked, and navy)	Sardines
Bok choy	Sesame seeds
Brazil nuts	Shrimp
Broccoli	Soy milk
Canned salmon	Soy nuts
Collard greens	Soybeans
Dried figs	Tahini paste
Edamame	Tempeh
Fortified orange juice	Tofu
Kale	Turnip greens

If that isn't enough to convince you that you won't feel deprived on a dairy-free diet, turn the page. The rest of this book is chock full of mouthwatering recipes to get you started on a dairy-free path.

The Least You Need to Know

◆ A clean and well-organized kitchen is important, especially when dealing with milk allergy.

◆ In addition to soy products, numerous nondairy milk alternatives and delicious substitutions are available for dairy-free cooking.

◆ Easy techniques and some unexpected ingredients assist you in creating consistency and flavor as you cook without milk.

◆ Nutritional concerns and calcium intake are easily addressed and resolved, thanks to some unexpected nutrition sources—all dairy free.

Part 2 Fresh Starts

Starting your day the dairy-free way might present a few dilemmas to the die-hard coffee-with-cream, buttered-toast, and milk-soaked-cereal diners among you. After all, isn't dairy in some form always the essential member of any proper breakfast table? Not necessarily.

In Part 2, you're introduced to some amazing breakfast foods that don't contain a drop of cow's milk. From quick weekday breakfast treats like hot cereal and bacon and egg wraps, to terrific brunch dishes you can make when you have a little more time, the dairy-free breakfasts in Part 2 will delight you. And yes, they're all made without milk, butter, and even cheese.

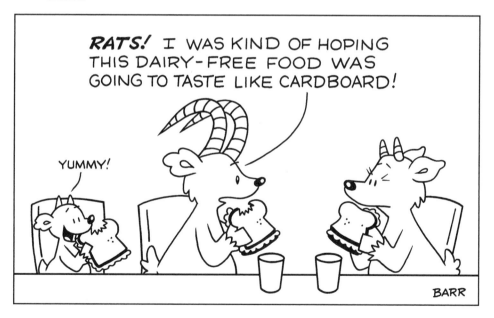

Chapter 3

Hot and Cold Beverages

In This Chapter

- ◆ Cups of creamy, warm comfort
- ◆ Rich, dairy-free solutions
- ◆ Smooth-as-silk smoothies

If you think that by eliminating dairy you'll be left with flavorless, watered-down drinks, think again. Cow's milk has no claim on rich and creamy! From popular lattes to chai and hot cocoa, many soy-based products as well as super-flavorful nut and grain milks can step in to satisfy your desire for richness and replicate the role the usual milk and cream might play. If cool and creamy is your goal, dairy-free frozen ices and yogurts combine with fresh fruit for the smoothest and tastiest refreshments around, and discerning taste buds will find it hard to resist the surprisingly rich and alluring dairy-free treats in this chapter.

So put down the milk carton, and start whipping up some of the best beverage selections you'll ever make! In this chapter, you discover the wonderful variety of ways to re-create your favorite milk-laden beverages with dynamic and delicious substitutes.

Café Non Latte

Creamy and delicious latte without milk? Mais oui, mon ami!
Flavorful vanilla soy milk steps in for a rich and yummy result.

Yield: 2 servings
Prep time: 3 minutes
Cook time: 3 minutes
Serving size: 1 cup

1 cup vanilla soy milk   **Dash ground cinnamon**

1 cup hot brewed coffee

1. In a small saucepan over medium heat, whisk vanilla soy milk
   for about 3 minutes or until steamy hot and frothy.

2. Divide coffee between 2 mugs, and whisk ½ of soy milk into
   each. Top with ground cinnamon, and serve immediately.

 Dairy Don't _____

Products labeled "nondairy creamers" may contain sodium
caseinate, a milk derivative. Although this is fine for lactose-
intolerant coffee drinkers, those with milk allergies should steer
clear of such products.

Mocha Dream

Delectably fragrant chocolate almond milk makes this hot coffee drink truly delightful and dreamy.

1 cup chocolate almond milk	Dash cocoa powder
1 cup hot brewed coffee	

Yield: 2 servings
Prep time: 3 minutes
Cook time: 3 minutes
Serving size: 1 cup

1. In a small saucepan over medium heat, whisk chocolate almond milk for about 3 minutes or until steamy hot and frothy.

2. Divide coffee between 2 mugs and whisk ½ of chocolate almond milk into each. Top with cocoa powder, and serve immediately.

 Milk-Free Morsel _____

Keep a shaker of cocoa powder handy to add a quick boost of dairy-free chocolate flavor to hot drinks and desserts.

Green Tea Chai

Creamy rice milk infused with exotic spices highlights this sweet green tea version of the classic Indian hot drink.

Yield: 2 servings
Prep time: 10 minutes
Cook time: 5 minutes
Serving size: 1 cup

1 cup rice milk

2 TB. light brown sugar

1 cinnamon stick

4 cardamom pods, lightly crushed

2 whole cloves

3 black peppercorns

1 cup strongly brewed green tea

1. In a small saucepan, combine rice milk, light brown sugar, cinnamon stick, cardamom pods, cloves, and peppercorns.

2. Place the pan over medium heat, and whisking occasionally, cook for 5 minutes or until sugar dissolves and mixture begins to boil. Remove from heat and allow to sit for 10 minutes.

3. Strain rice milk mixture through a fine sieve into a clean saucepan, and stir in green tea. Heat to just boiling.

4. Divide between 2 mugs, and serve immediately.

 Free Fact

Unlike almond milk, rice milk does not contain a significant amount of calcium, but commercial brands are often calcium-fortified for a boost of this essential mineral.

Almond Honey Tea

The wonderful aroma and flavor of almonds is enhanced with sweet almond milk and a spoonful of luscious honey in this unusual hot tea delight.

½ cup water	1 almond flavored teabag
½ cup vanilla almond milk	1 TB. honey

Yield: 1 serving
Prep time: 2 minutes
Cook time: 5 minutes
Serving size: 1 cup

1. In a small saucepan combine water and vanilla almond milk.

2. Place over high heat and bring to a boil. Remove from heat, add teabag to the saucepan, and steep for 5 minutes.

3. To serve, remove teabag, pour mixture into a mug, and stir in honey.

Dairy Don't _____

Look for the addition of gluten in flavored teas if this allergy is also one you need to watch.

Steamy, Creamy Hot Chocolate

A double whammy of deep, delicious chocolate along with soy creamer makes this amazing treat unbelievably rich and flavorful.

Yield: 2 servings
Prep time: 3 minutes
Cook time: 5 minutes
Serving size: 1 cup

1 cup chocolate soy milk

1 cup vanilla soy creamer

3 TB. cocoa powder

1 TB. sugar

Marshmallows

1. In a medium saucepan, combine chocolate soy milk, soy creamer, cocoa powder, and sugar.

2. Place the pan over medium heat, and whisking constantly, cook for about 5 minutes or until steamy hot and frothy.

3. Divide between 2 mugs, top with marshmallows, and serve immediately.

Lactose Lingo

Marshmallows are a popular confection made from sugar or corn syrup, water, gelatin, and flavorings. The gelatin, which is not vegan, mimics the sticky quality of the marshmallow plant that was used as an ingredient in original recipes.

Chocolate-Almond Cocoa Delight

Nutty and fragrant chocolate almond milk combines with rich and tropical coconut cream to create this superb-tasting hot beverage sure to delight all who try it.

2 cups chocolate almond milk	⅓ cup coconut cream, chilled
1 tsp. orgeat or almond syrup	2 TB. confectioners' sugar
1 TB. cocoa powder	1 tsp. sliced almonds (optional)

Yield: 2 servings
Prep time: 5 minutes
Cook time: 3 minutes
Serving size: 1 cup

1. In a small saucepan over medium heat, whisk together chocolate almond milk, orgeat syrup, and cocoa powder for about 3 minutes or until steamy hot and frothy. Transfer to a back burner and keep warm over low heat.

2. In a small bowl, combine coconut cream and confectioners' sugar, and beat with an electric mixer on high speed for about 2 minutes or until soft peaks form.

3. Divide hot chocolate almond mixture between 2 mugs, and top each with a generous dollop of whipped coconut cream. Sprinkle with sliced almonds (if using), and serve immediately.

Milk-Free Morsel

Coconut cream is an excellent nondairy substitute for heavy whipping cream and can be used in recipes that call for heavy cream. For whipping, be sure it's well chilled so it will hold soft peaks.

Caramel Queen Frappé

Creamy and cool with a hint of coffee and sweetly decadent caramel, this frappé will fool any dairy lover's taste buds into believing it's the real thing.

Yield: 1 serving	
Prep time: 4 minutes	
Serving size: about 2 cups	

½ **cup cold coffee**

1 cup vanilla nondairy frozen dessert

½ **cup ice cubes**

2 TB. caramel syrup

1. In a blender, add coffee, nondairy frozen dessert, ice cubes, and caramel syrup, and blend until smooth.

2. Pour into a large tumbler, and serve immediately.

 Dairy Don't

Not all coffee bar syrups are completely dairy free or gluten-free. "Caramel syrup" versions are often safer than "caramel sauce." Always read labels carefully.

Banilla Shake-Up

This delicious combo of sweet banana and aromatic vanilla is a smooth and satisfying shake for every sweet-treat-seeker.

1 ripe medium banana, peeled and cut into chunks

½ cup ice cubes

½ cup vanilla nondairy frozen dessert

½ tsp. vanilla extract

Yield: 1 serving
Prep time: 4 minutes
Serving size: about 2 cups

1. In a blender, add banana, ice cubes, nondairy frozen dessert, and vanilla extract, and blend until smooth.

2. Pour into a large tumbler, and serve immediately.

 Milk-Free Morsel _____

Keep chunks of ripe bananas and other fresh fruit in a zipper-lock bag in the freezer for quick shake- and smoothie-making without the need for ice.

Chocolate-Soy Shake

This rich and intense chocolate dairy-free shake will become a staple for when the chocolate craving hits.

Yield: 1 serving
Prep time: 4 minutes
Serving size: about 2 cups

½ cup chocolate soy milk

1 cup chocolate nondairy frozen dessert

½ cup ice cubes

2 TB. cocoa powder

2 TB. sugar

1. In a blender, add chocolate soy milk, nondairy frozen dessert, ice cubes, cocoa powder, and sugar, and blend until smooth.

2. Pour into a large tumbler, and serve immediately.

Free Fact

A variety of nondairy frozen desserts can take the place of ice cream and are not soy based. Rice-, oat-, and coconut milk–based ices are a few options available in your supermarket or health food store.

Peanut Butter Cup

This sweet and tantalizing treat that's fit for slurping features the heavenly combination of chocolate and peanut butter.

Yield: 1 serving
Prep time: 5 minutes
Serving size: about 1½ cups

1 cup chocolate soy milk

½ cup frozen banana pieces

1 TB. cocoa powder

1 TB. honey

3 TB. smooth peanut butter

1. In a blender add chocolate soy milk, banana pieces, cocoa powder, honey, and peanut butter. Purée until smooth.

2. Pour into a tumbler and serve immediately.

 Dairy Don't _____

Although chocolate and nuts are always tasty combinations, be aware that popular chocolate hazelnut spreads contain dairy.

Berry Nice Smoothie

Who doesn't love the tangy sweetness of fresh berries in smoothies and summer desserts? Here a trio of succulent berries highlights this healthy and satisfying creamy-rich smoothie.

Yield: 1 serving
Prep time: 10 minutes
Serving size: about 2 cups

1 cup mixed fresh berries (strawberries, blueberries, and raspberries), washed and stemmed

1 cup strawberry soy yogurt

½ cup ice cubes

¼ cup vanilla soy milk

1 TB. strawberry syrup

1. In a blender, add berries, soy yogurt, ice cubes, vanilla soy milk, and strawberry syrup, and blend until smooth.

2. Pour into a large tumbler, and serve immediately.

Milk-Free Morsel

When fresh berries are costly or hard to find, use frozen mixed berries without syrup for your smoothies instead. Add them straight from the freezer, and you eliminate the need for ice.

Peachy Keen Smoothie

Sweet peach nectar and fruit highlight this creamy concoction guaranteed to satisfy an anytime urge for a slurp of summer flavor.

½ **cup peach nectar, well chilled**

⅔ **cup frozen peach slices**

½ **cup vanilla soy yogurt**

Yield: 1 serving
Prep time: 5 minutes
Serving size: about 1½ cups

1. In a blender add peach nectar, frozen peach slices, and vanilla soy yogurt. Blend until smooth.

2. Pour into a tumbler and serve immediately.

Free Fact _____

Yellow-fleshed peaches, the most popular in the United States, are more acidic than white peaches and slightly less sweet.

Mango-Tango Smoothie

Sweet and delicious tropical mango takes center stage in this refreshing drink that's terrific with food or on its own.

Yield: 1 serving
Prep time: 10 minutes
Serving size: about 1½ cups

1 ripe mango, peeled, pitted, diced, and frozen, or 1 cup frozen mango pieces

½ cup orange or pineapple juice

1 TB. honey

1. In a blender, add mango, orange juice, and honey, and blend until smooth.

2. Pour into a tall tumbler, and serve immediately.

🚫 **Dairy Don't** _____

Smoothies made strictly from fruit and their juices are always good dairy-free choices for refreshing beverages. Watch for purchased versions, however, which may contain cow's milk yogurt or whey powder, particularly if you have milk allergies.

Quick and Easy Breakfasts

In This Chapter

- Hot and creamy morning cereals
- Clever uses for dairy substitutes
- Quick, protein-packed egg dishes

Nothing's better on a cold morning than a bowl of piping-hot oatmeal, mixed-grain cereal, or cream of rice. But making these nourishing cereals dairy free can pose a challenge. Not anymore! In this chapter, you find terrific recipes for the creamiest of hot cereals that use a variety of faux milk products to add both richness and flavor.

Dairy substitutes are particularly handy at breakfast, so be sure to have a good supply of alternative milks, creamers, and margarine on hand. Many high-quality dairy-free margarines are available without trans fats and offer terrific buttery flavor.

And we haven't forgotten about eggs. From creamy scrambled eggs to a fast, no-flip frittata, we've got several protein-packed egg dishes in the following pages. So grab your apron! You're about to become a short-order cook!

Creamy Vanilla-Nut Oatmeal

Doubly delicious with two shots of fragrant vanilla, this quick and creamy oatmeal has a crunchy sugary-nut topping for added pizzazz.

Yield: 2 servings
Prep time: 5 minutes
Cook time: 7 minutes
Serving size: about ¼ cup

1 cup vanilla soy milk

⅓ cup water

½ tsp. vanilla extract

⅔ cup old-fashioned oats

Pinch salt

¼ cup chopped walnuts or almonds

1 TB. light brown sugar

1. In a medium saucepan over high heat, combine vanilla soy milk and water. Bring to a boil, and stir in vanilla extract, oats, and salt.

2. Bring mixture back to a boil, reduce heat to low, and cook, stirring often, for 5 minutes or until thickened. Remove from heat.

3. In a small bowl, stir together chopped walnuts or almonds and brown sugar. Divide cooked oatmeal between 2 serving bowls, top each with nut mixture, and serve.

 Milk-Free Morsel

Make a large batch of the sugar-nut topping ahead and store in the pantry for even quicker breakfast production. Use as a topping for dairy-free "ice creams" and yogurts as well.

Apple Pie Oatmeal

Aromatic prepared *apple pie spice* makes this delicious recipe a snap to create and a pleasure to enjoy.

1 cup water

⅓ cup apple juice

⅔ cup old-fashioned oats

Pinch salt

½ tsp. apple pie spice

1 medium yellow delicious apple, cored and diced small

2 heaping tsp. brown sugar

½ cup vanilla soy milk

Yield: 2 servings
Prep time: 4 minutes
Cook time: 7 minutes
Serving size: about 1 cup

1. In a medium saucepan over high heat bring water and apple juice to a boil. Stir in oats, salt, and apple pie spice.

2. Bring the mixture back to a boil, reduce heat to low, and cook, stirring often, for 3 minutes. Stir in diced apple and cook, continuing to stir often, for another 2 minutes until thickened.

3. Divide oatmeal between two serving bowls, top each with a teaspoon of brown sugar and pour half the vanilla soy milk around the edge of each. Serve immediately.

Lactose Lingo

Apple pie spice is a prepared spice mixture of cinnamon, nutmeg, and mace and can be found in the spice aisle of your supermarket.

Multigrain Breakfast Bowl

Chewy and satisfying, this flavorful blend of quick-cooking grains, finished off with rich creamer and sweet honey, is a welcome delight on a chilly morning.

Yield: 1 serving	
Prep time: 2 minutes	
Cook time: 3 minutes	
Serving size: about ¾ cup	

½ **cup multigrain hot cereal (rye, barley, oats, and wheat)**

½ **cup water**

½ **cup** *oat milk* **or water**

Pinch salt

2 TB. soy creamer

1 TB. honey

1. In a microwave-safe bowl, combine multigrain cereal, water, oat milk, and salt. Microwave on high for 2 or 3 minutes. Stir again and let stand for 2 minutes to thicken.

2. Transfer mixture to a serving bowl, pour soy creamer around the edge, drizzle honey on top, and serve.

Lactose Lingo _____

Oat milk is made from oat groats, water, and sometimes other grains or beans. Lightly textured and mildly flavored, it's a good dairy-free substitute for reduced-fat or skim milk.

Kicked Up Creamy Oat Bran

Thick, creamy, and fiber-rich as well, this scrumptious and satisfying cereal has all the sweet flavor of a just baked banana-nut and oat bran muffin.

1 cup vanilla soy milk

½ cup water

½ oat bran

Pinch salt

⅛ tsp. ground cinnamon

1 small banana, peeled and diced small

⅓ cup roughly chopped walnuts

1 heaping TB. brown sugar

Yield: 2 servings
Prep time: 3 minutes
Cook time: 7 minutes
Serving size: about 1 cup

1. In a medium saucepan combine vanilla soy milk and water and bring to a boil over high heat.

2. Stir in oat bran, salt, and cinnamon, return to boil, reduce heat to low, and cook, stirring often, for 4 minutes. Add diced banana and continue to cook, stirring often, until thickened, about 1 minute more.

3. In a small bowl combine walnuts and brown sugar.

4. Divide the cooked oat bran between two serving bowls and top each with half the walnut-sugar mixture. Serve immediately.

 Milk-Free Morsel

Consider replacing brown sugar with raw sugar when called for in cereals for added sparkle and crunch.

Cinnamon-Raisin Cream of Rice

Practically dessert for breakfast, this puddinglike bowl of creamy rice with the alluring aroma of cinnamon and the succulence of sweet raisins will be requested on a regular basis.

Yield: 1 serving
Prep time: 3 minutes
Cook time: 2 minutes
Serving size: about 1 cup

1 cup rice milk	**1 tsp. sugar**
Dash salt	**¼ tsp. ground cinnamon**
¼ cup cream of rice cereal	**1½ TB. raisins**

1. In a medium saucepan over high heat, bring rice milk to a boil. Whisk in salt and cream of rice cereal, and return to a boil. Reduce heat to low, and simmer for 30 seconds, whisking constantly.

2. Remove from heat and stir in sugar, cinnamon, and raisins. Cover and let stand for 1 minute to thicken.

3. Transfer to a bowl and serve immediately.

Free Fact

Rice milk is usually made from brown rice, not white rice. Unsweetened rice milk actually has a hint of natural sweetness due to the breakdown of carbohydrates into sugars during the milk-making process.

Make-Ahead Maple-Pecan Granola

Have this delicious maple-flavor homemade granola on hand for a
quick morning treat with your choice of milk substitute.

2½ cups old-fashioned oats	**¼ cup light brown sugar**
3 TB. *sesame seeds*	**Pinch salt**
¼ cup vegetable oil	**½ cup roughly chopped pecans**
¼ cup maple syrup	

Yield: 6 servings
Prep time: 10 minutes
Cook time: 30 minutes
Serving size: ½ cup

1. Preheat the oven to 325°F.

2. In a medium mixing bowl, combine oats and sesame seeds.

3. In a small saucepan over medium heat, combine vegetable oil,
   maple syrup, brown sugar, and salt, and simmer, stirring often,
   for 2 or 3 minutes or until sugar has dissolved. Remove from
   heat, pour over oat mixture, and stir well to coat.

4. Transfer mixture to a large baking sheet with a rim and spread
   out evenly. Bake for 20 to 25 minutes or until golden and crisp,
   occasionally shaking the pan to evenly brown.

5. Remove from the oven, and stir in pecans.

6. Allow to cool completely, and store in an airtight container for
   up to 3 weeks.

Lactose Lingo

Sesame seeds, also called *benne,* derive from the sesame
plant and have been used in cooking and oil-making for centu-
ries. They are a great source of calcium and may help reduce
cholesterol when eaten regularly. Some people are allergic to
sesame, so ask before serving.

Egg-Cellent Scramble

It's all in the wrist in this slow-stirred, super-creamy, dairy-free egg scramble. Margarine adds buttery flavor, while a pinch nutritional yeast flakes contribute a tasty hint of cheese.

Yield: 1 serving	
Prep time: 3 minutes	
Cook time: 3 minutes	
Serving size: 2 eggs	

1 TB. dairy-free margarine	Pinch nutritional yeast flakes
2 large eggs	Salt and pepper
2 TB. water	

1. In medium nonstick skillet over medium-low heat, melt margarine, swirling to coat the bottom of the pan.

2. In a small mixing bowl, whisk together eggs, water, nutritional yeast flakes, salt, and pepper. Pour into the skillet and, using a wooden spoon, constantly and gently stir, working from the edge of the pan into the center.

3. Cook for 1 or 2 minutes or until eggs are thickened but still moist, and transfer to a warm plate. Serve immediately.

🚫 **Dairy Don't** _____

Clarified butter or ghee may contain lingering milk solids, so avoid these if you have milk allergies. However, butter may not be off-limits if you're lactose intolerant, as it contains very little lactose. Check with your doctor before deciding whether butter in any form is okay for you.

French Herb Omelet

Heavenly fragrant herbes de Provence, featuring savory aromatic herbs, highlights this soft and moist omelet that's as easy to make as it is delicious.

1 TB. dairy-free margarine	Salt and pepper
2 large eggs	1 tsp. herbes de Provence
3 TB. soy milk	

Yield: 1 serving
Prep time: 2 minutes
Cook time: 4 minutes
Serving size: 1 omelet

1. In a medium nonstick skillet over medium-low heat, melt margarine, swirling to coat the bottom of the pan.

2. In a small mixing bowl, whisk together eggs, soy milk, salt, pepper, and herbes de Provence. Pour into the skillet and, using a wooden spoon, gently stir for 30 seconds.

3. Cover the skillet, reduce heat to low, and cook for 1 more minute or until eggs are almost set.

4. Crumble herbes de Provence with your fingers evenly over egg surface, and continue to cook, covered, for 1 more minute.

5. Remove the lid, and using a large spatula, carefully fold ⅓ of omelet toward the center. Repeat on the other side. Transfer to a plate, and serve immediately.

Lactose Lingo

Herbes de Provence is a dried herb blend typically consisting of rosemary, marjoram, basil, bay leaf, thyme, and lavender. It reflects the culinary flavors of France's Provence region.

No-Flip Potato Frittata

Fruity olive oil eliminates the need for butter in this hearty egg breakfast that combines the Mediterranean scent of oregano with buttery-flavored Yukon gold potatoes.

Yield: 2 servings

Prep time: 7 minutes

Cook time: 13 minutes

Serving size: ½ frittata

2 TB. olive oil

1 medium Yukon gold potato, boiled, peeled, and cut into ¼-in.-thick slices

¼ tsp. garlic powder

Salt and pepper

1 tsp. dried oregano

4 large eggs, beaten

1. In a medium nonstick skillet over medium heat, heat olive oil. Add potato slices in a single layer in the bottom of the skillet, and sprinkle with garlic powder, salt, pepper, and dried oregano. Fry potatoes for about 1 minute or until lightly browned. Flip potatoes over and fry 1 more minute.

2. Pour in beaten eggs, cover, and cook for about 10 minutes or until eggs are set but still runny on top. Check occasionally to be sure frittata is not browning too quickly on the bottom, and reduce heat if necessary.

3. Remove the skillet from heat and place under a preheated broiler for 1 minute to finish cooking the top, moving the skillet around to cook evenly.

4. Loosen edges of frittata with a knife, and using a spatula, slide it onto a warm platter. Serve immediately.

Milk-Free Morsel

If your skillet doesn't have an oven-proof handle, wrap a few layers of aluminum foil around the handle to protect it while broiling. Be sure to grab it with an oven mitt on!

Ham-It-Up Eggs on Toast

Smoky and flavorful Canadian bacon kicks up egg on toast for a hearty, nutritious, and quick breakfast.

1 tsp. vegetable oil	1 slice whole-grain bread, toasted
1 slice Canadian bacon	
1 large egg	½ tsp. chopped fresh parsley
Salt and pepper	

Yield: 1 serving
Prep time: 2 minutes
Cook time: 4 minutes
Serving size: 1 egg on toast

1. In a medium nonstick skillet over medium heat, heat vegetable oil. Add bacon and cook for about 1 minute or until lightly brown. Flip bacon over and cook 1 more minute.

2. Move bacon to one side of the skillet, and crack egg on the other side. Sprinkle egg with salt and pepper, cover skillet, reduce heat to low, and cook for 1 or 2 minutes or until egg white is firm and yolk is opaque.

3. Place warm toast on a serving plate, and using a spatula, place cooked egg on top of bacon and transfer both to toast. Sprinkle with chopped parsley, and serve immediately.

⊘ Dairy Don't

Some whole-grain breads may contain nuts, so be sure to read labels carefully if nut allergies are a concern. Substitute whole-wheat or white bread if in doubt, and always check the label.

Bacon and Egg Burrito

Crispy, delicious bacon strips add flavor to a quick-scrambled egg for a tangy, Mexican-style breakfast treat.

Yield: 1 serving	
Prep time: 2 minutes	
Cook time: 5 minutes	
Serving size: 1 burrito	

3 strips bacon	Dash chili powder
1 large egg	1 burrito-size flour tortilla, warmed
Pinch ground black pepper	1 TB. salsa

1. In a medium nonstick skillet over medium-high heat, fry bacon strips for about 3 minutes or until crispy.

2. Transfer bacon to a paper towel to drain, and pour off all but 1 teaspoon bacon drippings from the skillet.

3. Reduce heat to medium, and crack egg into the skillet. Cook, stirring frequently, for about 1 minute or until scrambled. Season with pepper and chili powder, and scoop egg into the center of tortilla.

4. Place cooked bacon on top of egg, add salsa, and fold up, burrito style. Serve immediately.

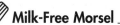

Milk-Free Morsel

No time to fry? Cook bacon strips the night before and store in the refrigerator. Reheat on a paper towel in the microwave for 15 to 30 seconds.

Quick Egg-and-Cheese Muffin

You'll never go back to traditional poaching after you taste the result of this delicious "cheesy" English muffin breakfast treat.

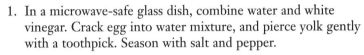

⅓ cup water

⅛ tsp. white vinegar

1 large egg

Salt and pepper

1 English muffin, split and toasted

1 slice nondairy American cheese

Yield: 1 serving		
Prep time: 2 minutes		
Cook time: 3 minutes		
Serving size: 1 egg muffin		

1. In a microwave-safe glass dish, combine water and white vinegar. Crack egg into water mixture, and pierce yolk gently with a toothpick. Season with salt and pepper.

2. Cover loosely with a paper towel, and microwave on high for 1 or 2 minutes. Remove egg with a slotted spoon, and place on 1 muffin half.

3. Place cheese on other muffin half, and microwave on high for 15 to 30 seconds to melt cheese.

4. Top egg half with cheese half, and serve immediately.

Free Fact

The vinegar in the poaching water keeps the egg white from dispersing and creating "threads." It's all pretty scientific, but in a nutshell, the vinegar lowers the surface tension of the water, enabling the white to cook quicker before it has a chance to spread out.

Chapter 5

Weekend Brunch Delights

In This Chapter

- ◆ Pancakes, hot off the griddle
- ◆ Egg-cellent brunch ideas
- ◆ Marvelous muffins and breads

On weekends, we usually have the luxury of a bit more time to create more substantial breakfasts or brunches. And good news! Many favorites such as pancakes and waffles can be easily adapted to a dairy-free diet. That's where this chapter comes in.

In addition to substituting with soy or other dairy-free milks and margarine, using some unusual ingredients can really jazz up griddle favorites with terrific flavor, texture, and moistness. And when it comes to some classic egg brunch dishes like eggs Benedict or a quiche, you'll no longer have to sacrifice flavor or tradition, thanks to the easy and creative versions in this chapter. As for irresistible muffins and brunch breads, you'll be the expert in the kitchen as you create treats whose wafting aroma of baked goodness will bring everyone to the table as fast as they can manage.

After trying some of the recipes in this chapter, you'll see that dairy-free brunch will never lack excitement again, and no one in your house will want to sleep in and risk missing your special weekend creations.

Silver-Dollar Pancakes

Light and fluffy with a "buttery" taste, these little delights will be gobbled up faster than you can make them.

Yield: *6 servings*
Prep time: 25 minutes
Cook time: 10 minutes
Serving size: 6 pancakes

1 cup all-purpose flour	**1 large egg, slightly beaten**
1 TB. sugar	**1 cup soy or rice milk**
2 tsp. baking powder	**2 TB. dairy-free margarine, melted**
¼ tsp. salt	

1. In a medium mixing bowl, whisk together flour, sugar, baking powder, and salt.

2. In another medium bowl, combine egg, soy milk, and melted margarine. Add wet ingredients to flour mixture, and stir just to combine without overmixing. Set aside for 15 minutes.

3. Heat a large griddle over medium heat, and coat with a little vegetable oil.

4. For each pancake, pour 1 tablespoon batter onto hot griddle. When bubbles begin to form, turn pancakes over and cook for about 3 minutes total or until lightly golden. Repeat with remaining batter, adding more oil to the griddle as necessary. Keep warm on a heated platter covered with foil or serve immediately.

Free Fact

Silver-dollar pancakes were named after the coins they resemble, first minted in Philadelphia in 1794, and kept in circulation until 1965.

Fluffy Whole-Wheat Pancakes

Satisfying and delicious with the flavor of vanilla and a hint of
cinnamon, these nutritious pancakes will become a regular weekend
request.

½ cup whole-wheat flour	¼ tsp. ground cinnamon
½ cup all-purpose flour	1 cup vanilla soy milk
2 tsp. baking powder	2 large eggs, slightly beaten
¼ tsp. salt	1 TB. vegetable oil

Yield: 4 servings

Prep time: 20 minutes
Cook time: 15 minutes
Serving size: 2 pancakes

1. In a medium mixing bowl, whisk together whole-wheat flour,
   all-purpose flour, baking powder, salt, and cinnamon.

2. In another medium bowl, whisk together vanilla soy milk,
   eggs, and vegetable oil. Add wet ingredients to flour mixture,
   and stir just to combine without overmixing. Set aside for
   10 minutes.

3. Heat a large griddle over medium heat, and coat with a little
   vegetable oil.

4. Spoon batter onto the griddle to make 3- or 4-inch-wide
   pancakes. Cook for 1 or 2 minutes per side or until golden.
   Keep warm on a heated platter covered with foil or serve
   immediately.

Milk-Free Morsel

Leftover weekend pancakes make for a quick weekday
breakfast with a short zap in the microwave. Simply heat 1 or 2
pancakes uncovered on a serving plate for 1 minute on high. To
store, wrap the leftover cakes in plastic and refrigerate to keep
them fresh.

Chocolate-Chocolate-Chip Pancakes

Doubly delicious chocolatey pancakes get an added flavor boost from chocolate soy milk for a sweet beginning to weekend fun.

Yield: 4 servings
Prep time: 15 minutes
Cook time: 15 minutes
Serving size: 2 pancakes

1 cup all-purpose flour

2 TB. cocoa powder

2 TB. sugar

2 tsp. baking powder

¼ tsp. salt

1¼ cups chocolate soy milk

2 large eggs, slightly beaten

½ tsp. vanilla extract

1 TB. dairy-free margarine, melted

⅔ cup dairy-free chocolate chips

1. In a medium mixing bowl, whisk together flour, cocoa powder, sugar, baking powder, and salt.

2. In another medium bowl, whisk together chocolate soy milk, eggs, vanilla extract, and melted margarine. Add wet ingredients to flour mixture, and stir just to combine without overmixing. Set aside for 10 minutes.

3. Heat a large griddle over medium heat, and coat with a little vegetable oil.

4. Pour batter onto the hot griddle to form 3- or 4-inch-wide pancakes, and sprinkle evenly with chocolate chips. When batter begins to bubble, turn pancakes over and continue to cook for about 4 minutes total or until golden. Keep warm on a heated platter covered with foil or serve immediately.

 Milk-Free Morsel

These leftover pancakes would make a great dessert on any other day, topped, of course, with dairy-free ice cream!

Oven-Baked Vanilla-Soy French Toast

No need to drag out the griddle for this thick and hearty French toast that's full of delicious vanilla flavor, thanks to sweet vanilla soy milk.

4 large eggs

1 cup vanilla soy milk

½ tsp. ground cinnamon

8 (1-in.-thick) slices Texas toast or country-style bread

Yield: 4 servings
Prep time: 1 hour or overnight
Cook time: 15 minutes
Serving size: 2 slices

1. In a large mixing bowl, whisk together eggs, vanilla soy milk, and ground cinnamon.

2. Place bread in a 9×13-inch casserole dish, and evenly pour egg mixture over top. Turn slices to absorb liquid, cover, and refrigerate for 30 minutes or overnight.

3. Preheat the oven to 400°F. Coat a large baking sheet evenly with about 1 teaspoon margarine.

4. Place soaked bread slices in a single layer on the prepared baking sheet, and bake for 15 minutes or until golden brown, turning over slices halfway through. Remove from the oven and keep warm on a heated platter, or serve immediately.

Free Fact

Commercially sliced "Texas toast" is simply bread sliced at double the thickness, ideal for French toast recipes as well as for grilling.

Stuffed Strawberry French Toast

A rich and creamy surprise filling awaits in this sweet strawberry version of a classic breakfast that's almost like starting your day with dessert.

Yield: 2 servings

Prep time: 15 minutes
Cook time: 10 minutes
Serving size: 1 stuffed French toast

1 (8-oz.) container fresh strawberries, washed, hulled, and sliced

2 TB. sugar

4 slices white sandwich bread, crusts removed

4 TB. dairy-free cream cheese

1 large egg

1 large egg white

⅔ cup soy milk

1 TB. dairy-free margarine

1 TB. vegetable oil

Non-dairy topping (optional)

1. Set aside 12 strawberry slices. Combine remaining slices with sugar in a medium bowl, stir and set aside.

2. Place bread slices on a cutting board and spread each slice with 1 tablespoon. dairy-free cream cheese. Top two of the slices with the strawberries that were set aside, and place remaining bread slices on top, cream cheese sides together, to make two sandwiches.

3. In a shallow bowl, whisk together egg, egg white, and soy milk.

4. Melt together margarine and oil in a large nonstick skillet over medium heat.

5. Dip each sandwich into the egg mixture on both sides to moisten and carefully place in the skillet. Cook over medium heat for 3 to 4 minutes per side until lightly golden on the outside and warm on the inside.

6. Transfer each stuffed French toast to a serving plate, spoon the sugared strawberries and any accumulated juices over the French toast, and add a dollop of non-dairy topping, if using. Serve immediately.

⊘ **Dairy Don't** _____

Non-dairy toppings are not appropriate for those with milk allergy as they usually contain casein. They are fine, however, for those who are lactose-intolerant.

Crispy Peanut Butter and Jelly Waffles

The all-time favorite sandwich combo will become a favorite weekend breakfast with these fun-to-make and sweet-to-eat waffles.

1 cup whole-wheat flour

1 cup all-purpose flour

2 TB. sugar

4 tsp. baking powder

¼ tsp. salt

⅔ cup creamy peanut butter

2 large eggs

2 TB. vegetable oil

2 cups soy milk

½ cup grape jelly

Yield: 4 servings
Prep time: 15 minutes
Cook time: 20 minutes
Serving size: 2 waffles

1. In a medium mixing bowl, whisk together whole-wheat flour, all-purpose flour, sugar, baking powder, and salt.

2. In another bowl, using an electric mixer on medium-high speed, beat together peanut butter, eggs, vegetable oil, and soy milk. Add wet ingredients to flour mixture, and stir just to combine without overmixing. Set aside for 10 minutes.

3. Heat a waffle iron according to the manufacturer's instructions, and coat lightly with vegetable oil. Pour batter into waffle iron in batches, and cook for 3 or 4 minutes per batch or until crisp and golden.

4. To serve, spread grape jelly over 4 waffles, and top with remaining 4 waffles to make sandwich.

Free Fact

In the early twentieth century, peanut butter was considered quite a delicacy for upper-class restaurant patrons. The Vanity Fair tearoom had a popular Peanut Butter and Watercress Sandwich on its menu.

Toasty Oat-Banana Waffles

Sweet, ripe bananas dot these hearty oat waffles flavored with brown sugar and a hint of nutmeg and cinnamon.

○ ❦ ◎

Yield: 4 servings

Prep time: 25 minutes
Cook time: 15 minutes
Serving size: 2 waffles

1¼ cups oat milk

1 TB. cider vinegar

1 cup old-fashioned rolled oats

1 cup all-purpose flour

3 TB. light brown sugar, firmly packed

1 TB. baking powder

½ tsp. baking soda

¼ tsp. salt

¼ tsp. ground cinnamon

Dash ground nutmeg

2 large eggs

3 TB. dairy-free margarine, melted

2 medium, ripe bananas, peeled and diced

1. In a small bowl, stir together oat milk and cider vinegar, and set aside.

2. In a medium mixing bowl, whisk together rolled oats, flour, light brown sugar, baking powder, baking soda, salt, cinnamon, and nutmeg.

3. In another mixing bowl, beat together eggs, melted margarine, and oat milk mixture. Add wet ingredients to flour mixture, and stir to combine without overmixing. Fold in diced banana.

4. Heat a waffle iron according to the manufacturer's instructions, and coat lightly with vegetable oil. Spoon batter into waffle iron in batches, and cook for 3 or 4 minutes per batch or until crispy and golden. Keep warm on a heated platter or serve immediately.

Free Fact

Nutmeg has nothing to do with nuts and is actually a seed from a tropical fruit tree. It provides two spices: nutmeg itself and mace, from the inner lining. Both are very similar in taste.

Unbelievable Eggs Benedict

A fabulous faux hollandaise sauce and savory Canadian bacon bring to life this amazing brunch delight that's no longer off-limits.

4 large eggs

1 TB. white wine vinegar

Pinch salt

2 English muffins, split and toasted

4 slices Canadian bacon, warmed

½ batch Dairy-Free Hollandaise (recipe in Chapter 16), warmed

Dash paprika

Yield: 2 servings	
Prep time: 20 minutes	
Cook time: 5 minutes	
Serving size: 2 eggs	

1. Crack each egg into a separate small bowl or cup.

2. Fill a large skillet with 3 inches water, cover, and bring to a boil over high heat. Stir in white wine vinegar and salt, and carefully pour in eggs. Turn off heat, cover, and allow to cook for about 3 minutes or until eggs are just firm. Remove eggs with a slotted spoon, and drain on paper towels.

3. Place toasted muffin halves on a plate, and top each with 1 slice bacon. Place 1 poached egg on each muffin half, and drizzle Dairy-Free Hollandaise sauce over top. Finish with a dash of paprika, and serve immediately.

 Dairy Don't

Many commercial brands of English muffins contain dairy, so read labels carefully. In a pinch, eggs Benedict are just as delicious served on toasted bagel halves or wheat bread toast.

Crustless Breakfast Quiche

Light, fluffy, and terrific for reheating, this bottomless quiche is tops in the flavor department with the addition of sun-dried tomatoes and vegan Parmesan cheese.

Yield: 4 servings
Prep time: 15 minutes
Cook time: 15 to 20 minutes
Serving size: 1 (4×4-inch) square

2 TB. cornstarch

½ cup soy milk

½ cup soy creamer

2 large eggs

3 TB. vegan Parmesan cheese

¼ tsp. salt

Dash cayenne

¼ cup chopped sun-dried tomatoes, not oil-packed

1. Preheat the oven to 400°F. Lightly coat an 8×8-inch nonstick pan with dairy-free margarine.

2. In a medium mixing bowl, add cornstarch. Slowly whisk in soy milk and soy creamer until smooth. Add eggs, vegan Parmesan cheese, salt, and cayenne, and whisk well to combine.

3. Pour mixture into the prepared pan, and sprinkle chopped sun-dried tomatoes over evenly. Bake for 15 to 20 minutes or until top is lightly golden and a toothpick inserted in the center comes out clean.

4. Cut into 4 equal squares and serve immediately, or cool and refrigerate if desired.

 Milk-Free Morsel _____

Cornstarch can be a handy thickener in the dairy-free kitchen, replacing the usual combination of butter and flour or reduced cream sauces. It does need to be cooked to come to its full thickening power, however.

English "Cream" Scones

You'll find no dairy in these quintessential flaky and "buttery" British creations that are fun to bake and even more delicious to eat.

1½ cups self-rising flour

1 TB. sugar

Pinch salt

3 TB. dairy-free stick margarine, diced and slightly softened

⅔ cup soy creamer

Yield: 10 scones	
Prep time: 30 minutes	
Cook time: 12 to 15 minutes	
Serving size: 1 or 2 scones	

1. Preheat the oven to 425°F. Line a baking sheet with parchment paper.

2. In a medium mixing bowl, stir together self-rising flour, sugar, and salt. Add diced margarine and, using a fork or a pastry blender, work margarine into flour mixture until mixture is the consistency of sand.

3. Stir in soy creamer a bit at a time until a soft dough forms. Turn out dough onto a lightly floured cutting board.

4. Roll dough into a ¾-inch-thick circle. Using a biscuit cutter or a 2-inch-wide drinking glass dipped in flour, cut out circles and transfer carefully to the baking sheet. Reroll and cut as necessary to use up remaining dough.

5. Bake for 12 to 15 minutes or until scones are golden on top and a toothpick inserted in the center comes out clean. Transfer to a wire rack to cool slightly before serving.

Free Fact

In English circles, the term *cream scone* or *cream tea* refers to clotted cream, a thickened, unpasteurized cream that's spread on scones with preserves. Milk, not cream, is the usual ingredient in English scones and tea.

Apple Cake Muffins

Moist and delectable, these marvelous muffins flavored with almond and cinnamon and topped with crunchy nuts are terrific for a weekend brunch—or any time of day!

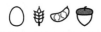

Yield: 12 muffins
Prep time: 25 minutes
Cook time: 25 to 30 minutes
Serving size: 1 or 2 muffins

1½ cups all-purpose flour

½ cup sugar

2 tsp. baking powder

½ tsp. plus ¼ tsp. ground cinnamon

¼ tsp. salt

1 cup grated, peeled, and cored raw apple (about 1 medium)

¼ cup (½ stick) dairy-free margarine, softened

1 large egg

½ cup almond milk

⅓ cup dark or light brown sugar, firmly packed

⅓ cup sliced almonds, slightly crumbled

1. Preheat the oven to 400°F. Line a regular 12-cup muffin pan with paper liners.

2. In a medium mixing bowl, whisk together flour, sugar, baking powder, ½ teaspoon cinnamon, and salt.

3. In another medium mixing bowl, and using an electric mixer on medium speed, beat together grated apple, margarine, egg, and almond milk just to combine. Stir in dry ingredients with a wooden spoon until just combined.

4. Fill the lined muffin tins ⅔ full.

5. In a small bowl, stir together brown sugar, almonds, and remaining ¼ teaspoon cinnamon. Sprinkle evenly over each muffin, and bake for 25 to 30 minutes or until lightly golden and a toothpick inserted in the center comes out clean.

6. Remove muffins from the oven and transfer to a wire rack to cool slightly before serving.

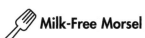

Milk-Free Morsel

Keep muffins moist for days by individually wrapping them in plastic and storing them in a tin or bread box.

Blueberry Crumb Muffins

Succulent blueberries burst with flavor in every mouthful while a crumbly topping adds another layer of sweetness and texture.

1¾ cup plus ½ cup all-purpose flour

½ cup sugar

2 tsp. baking powder

½ tsp. salt

Dash nutmeg

¾ cup soy milk

¼ cup vegetable oil

1 large egg

1 cup fresh blueberries, washed and stems removed

¼ cup (½ stick) dairy-free margarine

¼ cup firmly packed light brown sugar

Dash ground cinnamon

Confectioners' sugar

Yield: 12 muffins
Prep time: 20 minutes
Cook time: 20 to 25 minutes
Serving size: 1 or 2 muffins

1. Preheat the oven to 400°F. Line a regular 12-cup muffin pan with paper liners.

2. In a medium mixing bowl, whisk together 1¾ cups flour with sugar, baking powder, salt, and nutmeg.

3. In another medium mixing bowl, and using an electric mixer on medium speed, beat together soy milk, vegetable oil, and egg. Stir in dry ingredients with a wooden spoon until just combined. Fold in blueberries.

4. Fill lined muffin tins ⅔ full.

5. In a small bowl, using the back of a fork, combine margarine, remaining ½ cup flour, brown sugar, and cinnamon until crumbs form. Sprinkle evenly over each muffin, and bake for 20 to 25 minutes or until a toothpick inserted in the center comes out clean.

6. Remove muffins from the oven and transfer to a wire rack to cool slightly before removing from the tin. Cool completely and dust lightly with confectioners' sugar.

Milk-Free Morsel

For a year round supply of succulent fresh blueberries, spread them out on a baking sheet with a rim and put in the freezer. Transfer frozen berries to a Ziploc bag and store for up to 6 months.

Dairy-Free Corn Muffins

Deliciously moist straight from the oven or perfect for making cornbread stuffing, these tasty, not too sweet, muffins will become a regular habit at most every meal.

Yield: 12 muffins
Prep time: 10 minutes
Cook time: 20 to 25 minutes
Serving size: 1 or 2 muffins

1 cup *stone-ground cornmeal*

1 cup all-purpose flour

2 TB. sugar

1 TB. baking powder

1 tsp. salt

1 cup soy or oat milk

2 TB. dairy-free margarine, melted

2 large eggs, slightly beaten

1. Preheat the oven to 400°F. Lightly coat a regular 12-cup muffin tin with dairy-free margarine.

2. In a medium mixing bowl, whisk together cornmeal, flour, sugar, baking powder, and salt.

3. In another medium bowl, whisk together soy milk, melted margarine, and eggs. Add wet ingredients to flour mixture, and stir just to combine.

4. Pour batter into the prepared muffin tins ⅔ full, and bake for 20 to 25 minutes or until edges are golden and a toothpick inserted in the center comes out clean.

5. Remove muffins from the oven, and let rest for 5 minutes. Run a sharp knife around edges of muffins, remove from the pan, and transfer them to a wire rack to cool slightly before serving.

Lactose Lingo

Stone-ground cornmeal, as opposed to the more common steel ground, retains some of the hull and germ of the corn kernel, resulting in more flavor but a shorter shelf life. Store in the refrigerator for best results.

Banana Breakfast Bread

Nothing beats the sweet welcome of this cinnamon-scented banana bread as its enticing aroma wafts through the house.

½ cup vegetable oil	1½ cups all-purpose flour
¾ cup sugar	1 tsp. ground cinnamon
2 large eggs	1 tsp. baking powder
2 tsp. vanilla extract	½ tsp. baking soda
1½ cups mashed ripe bananas (about 2 medium)	¼ tsp. salt
	Dash ground nutmeg

Yield: 1 (9×5-inch) loaf

Prep time: 20 minutes

Cook time: 40 to 50 minutes

Serving size: 1 (1-inch-thick) slice

1. Preheat the oven to 350°F. Lightly coat a 9×5-inch loaf pan with dairy-free margarine and flour.

2. In a medium bowl, and using an electric mixer on medium speed, beat together vegetable oil, sugar, eggs, vanilla extract, and mashed bananas.

3. In another medium bowl, whisk together flour, cinnamon, baking powder, baking soda, salt, and nutmeg. Add dry ingredients to banana mixture in 3 batches, stirring just to combine each time.

4. Pour batter into the loaf pan, and bake for 40 to 50 minutes or until top is golden and a toothpick inserted in the center comes out clean.

5. Cool for 10 minutes in the pan, loosen the sides, and turn out, transferring to a wire rack to cool completely before slicing.

Milk-Free Morsel

Freeze browned bananas in their peel for bread and muffin baking later. Simply defrost them in the refrigerator, peel, and mash.

Part

Appetizers and Light Fare

If you're looking for sensational snacks and hors d'oeuvres, all made dairy free, you've definitely come to the right place. The innovative recipes in Part 3 demonstrate that dairy-free eating does not mean missing out on your favorites.

If soup and salad are what you're after, look no further. In the following chapters, you'll find an enticing array of satisfying soups and salads—including dairy-free dressings—that are perfect for lunch or even as the star of a light meal. And you thought dairy-free was going to be boring!

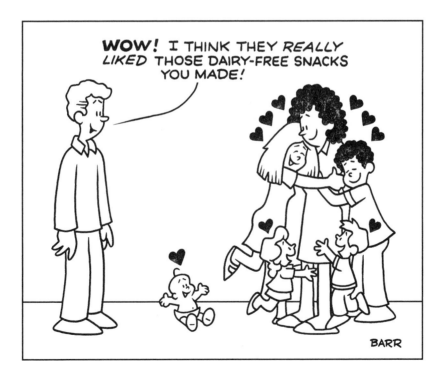

Easy Snacks and Sandwiches

In This Chapter

◆ New ways with appetizing favorites

◆ Sensational crispy nibbles

◆ Sandwiches that satisfy

You might be surprised to learn that many commercial snack products contain a variety of milk protein ingredients, often inconspicuously labeled. The delectable treats in this chapter help remove the worry from snacking. After sampling a few of the flavorful nibbles in this chapter, munchers will be far from disappointed!

Simple sandwiches can also hold a bit of uncertainty when it comes to hidden dairy. Having a few reliable selections in your repertoire will go far to quell any fears of accidental dairy intake. So start your snack- and sandwich-making, pronto! You'll be deliciously pleased you did.

Piglets in a Blanket

A quick dairy-free shortening dough is the perfect foil for juicy cocktail franks served with a tangy honey mustard dipping sauce.

Yield: 4 to 6 servings	
Prep time: 30 minutes	
Cook time: 20 minutes	
Serving size: 4 to 6 pieces	

2¼ cups flour

1 tsp. salt

1 tsp. sugar

¾ cup dairy-free shortening or margarine

2 or 3 TB. ice water

½ cup yellow mustard

3 TB. honey

24 cocktail beef franks

1. In a medium mixing bowl, whisk together flour, salt, and sugar. Using a fork or pastry blender, cut shortening into flour mixture until a grainy consistency is reached. Add enough ice water until dough holds together. Chill dough for 20 minutes.

2. Preheat the oven to 400°F. Line a baking sheet with parchment paper.

3. In a small serving dish, stir together yellow mustard and honey. Set aside.

4. Roll out dough on a floured surface to ⅛ inch thickness. Using a pizza cutter or large, sharp knife, cut into 24 squares, and wrap each square around a cocktail frank like a blanket. Place seam side down on the baking sheet.

5. Bake for 15 to 20 minutes or until pastry is golden. Serve with honey mustard dipping sauce.

Milk-Free Morsel

Freeze unbaked piglets on the lined baking sheet, transfer to a freezer bag, and bake from frozen in a preheated 350°F oven for 30 minutes.

Black Bean Nachos

These tempting nachos, with a good amount of protein and calcium, will keep them coming back for more. Add green chilies to the nacho sauce for heat lovers!

24 corn tortilla chips	2 TB. cornstarch
1 cup canned black beans, drained and rinsed	1 cup soy or rice milk
1 small ripe tomato, cored and diced	2 TB. tahini (sesame seed paste)
3 TB. diced red onion	1 tsp. lemon juice
⅓ cup nutritional yeast flakes	1 or 2 TB. canned diced green chiles (optional)
1 tsp. turmeric	Salt and pepper

> *Yield: 4 servings*
> **Prep time:** 20 minutes
> **Cook time:** 15 minutes
> **Serving size:** 6 nachos

1. On a large serving platter, arrange tortilla chips in a single layer. Top with black beans, tomato, and onion.

2. In a small saucepan, whisk together nutritional yeast flakes, turmeric, and cornstarch. Add soy milk, tahini, and lemon juice, and stir to combine.

3. Over medium heat, whisking often, bring sauce to a boil. Reduce heat to low, and continue whisking for 2 or 3 minutes or until sauce has thickened and is bubbly. Add chiles (if using), season with salt and pepper, and pour sauce over chips. Serve immediately.

 Milk-Free Morsel

Use this terrific nacho "cheese" sauce to top french fries, burgers, or other Mexican dishes where cheese is called for, such as enchiladas and burritos.

Chicken-Chile Quesadillas

Quick and hearty with a delicious filling, these quesadillas will become a part of your appetizer repertoire in no time. A dairy-free cream cheese filling holds it all together.

Yield: 2 servings

Prep time: 10 minutes

Cook time: 5 minutes

Serving size: ½ quesadilla

2 burrito-size flour tortillas	2 TB. canned diced green chiles
2 TB. dairy-free cream cheese	Pinch salt
⅔ cup diced cooked chicken breast	Dash ground cumin
	1 TB. vegetable oil

1. Lay tortillas on a flat work surface, and evenly spread 1 tablespoon cream cheese over each.

2. In a small bowl, gently combine chicken, chiles, salt, and cumin. Spoon mixture evenly over 1 tortilla, top with remaining tortilla, and press together firmly.

3. In a large, nonstick skillet over medium heat, heat vegetable oil. Add quesadilla and cook, pressing down gently with a metal spatula, for 2 or 3 minutes or until lightly golden. Flip over quesadilla, and continue to cook another 2 minutes or until browned and heated through.

4. Transfer quesadilla to a cutting board, and slice into 8 triangles. Serve immediately.

🚫 **Dairy Don't**

Not all soy-based cream cheese substitutes are whey free, so be sure to read labels carefully. Tofutti brand Better Than Cream Cheese is whey free.

Potato-Onion Tarts

These tasty tarts use thin-sliced potatoes as the crust, eliminating any dairy-free dough concerns. Sweet caramelized onions provide the filling, while a dollop of dairy-free sour cream and chives finish it off.

2 large Idaho potatoes, peeled and cut into ⅛-in. slices

Vegetable oil cooking spray

Salt and pepper

2 TB. olive oil

4 medium Vidalia onions, peeled, halved, and cut into ¼-in.-thick slices

1 tsp. sugar

2 garlic cloves, minced

½ tsp. dried thyme

¼ cup dairy-free sour cream

1 TB. chopped fresh chives

Yield: 6 servings
Prep time: 30 minutes
Cook time: 30 to 40 minutes
Serving size: 2 tarts

1. Preheat the oven to 400°F. Lightly coat a 12-cup muffin tin with vegetable oil cooking spray.

2. Line the bottom and sides of each muffin tin cup with potato slices, overlapping slightly and pressing together. Lightly spray potatoes with vegetable oil cooking spray, and season with salt and pepper. Bake for about 20 minutes or until crisp and golden.

3. Meanwhile, in a large, nonstick frying pan over medium-high heat, heat olive oil. Add onions, season with salt and pepper, and sprinkle with sugar. Cook, stirring often, for 15 to 20 minutes or until onions are soft and golden. Stir in garlic and thyme, cook for 2 more minutes, and remove from heat.

4. Carefully remove potato crusts from the muffin pan and place on a serving platter. Distribute onion mixture by spoonfuls into crusts and top each with 1 teaspoon dairy-free sour cream and some fresh chives. Serve immediately.

Free Fact

Vidalia onions, which hail from Georgia, are not the only sweet onions available. Walla Walla, grown in Oregon and Washington States, and Oso Sweet, grown in the Andean Mountains of Chile, can also be found in most supermarkets.

Butternut Squash Crostini

Sweet roasted butternut squash and savory nut butter combine for a fabulous crostini topping in this easy, yet impressive hors d'oeuvre.

Yield: 8 servings
Prep time: 15 minutes
Cook time: 30 minutes
Serving size: 3 crostini

2 cups peeled, seeded, and cubed butternut squash (about 1½ lb. whole)

1 TB. vegetable oil

Salt and pepper

Dash ground cinnamon

1 tsp. olive oil

4 shallots, peeled and finely chopped

¼ cup almond butter

1 french baguette, sliced diagonally into 24 pieces

Extra-virgin olive oil

¼ cup sliced almonds

1. Preheat the oven to 375°F.

2. In a roasting pan, toss together squash, vegetable oil, salt, pepper, and cinnamon. Roast in the oven, stirring occasionally, for about 25 minutes or until squash is tender and lightly browned. Transfer mixture to the bowl of a food processor fitted with a steel blade. Keep the oven on.

2. In a small skillet over medium-high heat, heat olive oil. Add shallots and cook, stirring often, for about 5 minutes or until shallots are soft and lightly brown. Add to the food processor bowl along with almond butter.

3. Process squash mixture and shallots for 1 minute or until smooth and creamy. Transfer mixture to a large mixing bowl, and season with additional salt and pepper, if necessary.

4. Place bread slices in a single layer on a baking sheet, and brush each with a little extra-virgin olive oil. Toast in the oven for 8 minutes or until lightly browned.

5. Spread a heaping spoonful of squash mixture on each bread slice, sprinkle with sliced almonds, and serve.

Free Fact

Almond butter ranks second, behind soy nut butter, on the list of calcium-containing nut butters. Just 1 tablespoon offers 43 milligrams calcium.

Sea Salt Saltines

Tired of store-bought crackers with hidden milk powder or whey? Whip up a batch of these delicious crispy crackers for snacking and spreads, and you may never go back to store-bought again.

2 cups flour	¾ cup soy or rice milk
1 tsp. salt	Water
1 tsp. sugar	Coarse sea salt
2 TB. dairy-free margarine	

Yield: 5 servings
Prep time: 15 minutes
Cook time: 25 minutes
Serving size: 8 crackers

1. In the bowl of a food processor fitted with a steel blade, add flour, salt, and sugar, and pulse for about 30 seconds or until just combined. Add margarine and pulse for 30 more seconds or until mixture is crumbly.

2. While the processor is running, pour in soy milk until dough forms a ball. Turn off the processor, remove dough, and flatten into a disc. Wrap dough in plastic, and refrigerate for 25 minutes.

3. Preheat the oven to 325°F.

4. Roll out dough on a floured surface to a ¹⁄₁₆ inch thickness. Use a pizza cutter to cut dough into 2×4-inch rectangles, and transfer crackers to an ungreased baking sheet. Lightly brush with water and sprinkle with coarse salt.

5. Bake for about 20 minutes or until crackers are lightly browned and crisp. Transfer to a wire rack to cool, and store in an airtight container for up to 1 week.

Free Fact

Saltines, also called soda crackers, date to the nineteenth century. True soda crackers contain baking soda and yeast and go through an elaborate leavening process. Today, *saltines* may refer to any type of crisp, salted cracker.

Herbed Cheese Straws

Perfect for snacking or dipping, these cheese-free cheese straws will satisfy any urge to crunch and munch with their salty, savory flavor.

Yield: 4 servings
Prep time: 15 minutes
Cook time: 18 minutes
Serving size: 3 straws

¼ **cup dairy-free margarine**

½ **cup vegan Parmesan cheese**

½ **cup whole-wheat pastry flour**

½ **tsp. dried Italian herb mix**

¼ **tsp. salt**

Dash cayenne

2 or 3 TB. water

1. Preheat the oven to 350°F. Line a baking sheet with parchment paper.

2. In a large mixing bowl and with an electric mixer on medium speed, beat together margarine and vegan Parmesan cheese for 1 minute or until smooth.

3. In a small bowl, whisk together flour, Italian herb mix, salt, and cayenne. Add flour mixture to margarine mixture, and beat to combine. Add water a little at a time until a soft dough forms.

4. Turn out dough onto a floured surface, and roll into a 6-inch square, ½ inch thick. Cut into 12 equal strips, and twist each strip to form a spiral. Transfer sticks to the prepared baking sheet, and bake for 15 to 18 minutes or until lightly browned. Cool on a wire rack, and store in an airtight container for up to 1 week.

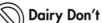 **Dairy Don't**

Some dry dairy-free cheese substitutes may have added ground nuts for flavor. Eat in the Raw's Parma! Vegan Parmesan, for example, contains organic walnuts. If nut allergies are a concern, stick to nutritional yeast flakes to mimic the flavor of cheese without fear of hidden nuts.

Movie Time Popcorn

Butter free with just a hint of oil and a dusting of exotic flavor, this delightfully delicious popcorn makes a terrific low-fat snack.

4 cups air-popped or stovetop homemade popcorn

Butter-flavored cooking spray

½ tsp. salt

¼ tsp. onion powder

¼ tsp. curry powder

¼ tsp. paprika

Yield: 4 servings	
Prep time: 5 minutes	
Serving size: 1 cup	

1. Spread warm popcorn on a baking sheet, and lightly coat with cooking spray.

2. Place salt, onion powder, curry powder, and paprika in a large zipper-lock bag, and shake to combine. Add coated popcorn to the bag, and shake well to distribute seasonings. Serve warm or at room temperature.

Free Fact

Buttered and flavored commercial popcorns, including microwave versions, can contain buttermilk, whey, and other milk products. Many butter "flavored" sprays, however, are completely dairy free.

Best-Ever Guacamole

Rich avocados provide the creamy consistency in this delicious guac that's not too spicy, but full of taste and tang.

Yield: 4 servings
Prep time: 15 minutes
Serving size: about ½ cup

2 ripe Hass avocados

Juice of ½ lime

½ small onion, finely chopped

2 ripe plum tomatoes, seeds removed and chopped

Dash hot pepper sauce

Salt and pepper

1. Slice avocados in half and twist apart. Remove seeds, and scoop out flesh into a medium mixing bowl. Add lime juice, and mash with the back of a fork or a potato masher.

2. Stir in onion, tomatoes, hot pepper sauce, salt, and pepper. Transfer to a dipping bowl, and serve immediately.

Variation: For **Mexican Five Layer Dip,** try this: in a shallow 1-quart bowl, spread 1 (15-ounce) can refried beans. Top with 1 cup prepared salsa and guacamole. Spread a thin layer of dairy-free sour cream on top, and sprinkle with shredded dairy-free cheddar cheese.

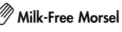 **Milk-Free Morsel**

Keep your guacamole looking fresh and green by placing a piece of paper towel saturated with lime juice directly on the surface. The acid from the lime juice will delay oxidation and browning.

Vidalia Onion Dip

Deliciously sweet Vidalia onions highlight this wonderfully creamy dip perfect for raw veggies or potato chips.

2 TB. dairy-free margarine	**8 oz. extra-firm tofu**
1 tsp. vegetable oil	**¼ tsp. garlic powder**
1 large Vidalia onion, peeled and minced	**½ tsp. prepared mustard**
	2 TB. nutritional yeast
Salt and pepper	

Yield: 4 to 6 servings

Prep time: 20 minutes

Cook time: 20 minutes

Serving size: about ¼ cup

1. Melt together margarine and vegetable oil in a large nonstick skillet over medium heat. Add minced onion and season with salt and pepper.

2. Cook the onions over medium heat, stirring occasionally, for about 20 minutes, until soft and just beginning to brown. Remove the skillet from the heat and set aside to cool.

3. Cut tofu into large chunks and place in the bowl of a food processor fitted with a steel blade. Add garlic powder, mustard, and nutritional yeast, and process for 1 to 2 minutes, until smooth and free of lumps.

4. Transfer the tofu to a mixing bowl and stir in the cooked onions. Taste for the addition of salt and pepper, and chill in the refrigerator for at least 30 minutes before serving.

Free Fact

Fresh tofu is generally sold as soft or silken, firm, and extra firm, depending upon the amount of water that has been drained and pressed from the block.

Creamy Spinach and Artichoke Dip

Amazingly dairy free, this favorite of hot dips gets its Mediterranean flavor from marinated artichokes and its creamy consistency from sweet, rich soy creamer.

Yield: 4 to 6 servings
Prep time: 15 minutes
Cook time: 12 minutes
Serving size: about ⅓ cup

1 TB. olive oil	Dash paprika
1 small onion, minced	1 cup frozen chopped spinach, cooked and squeezed dry
1 TB. all-purpose flour	
⅓ cup low-sodium chicken or vegetable broth	1 cup marinated artichokes, drained and chopped
1 cup soy creamer	2 TB. vegan Parmesan cheese

1. In a medium nonstick skillet over medium-high heat, heat olive oil. Add onion and cook, stirring often, for about 3 minutes or until onion is softened.

2. Stir in flour and cook, stirring often, for 1 or 2 more minutes.

3. Reduce heat to medium. Pour in chicken broth and soy creamer, add paprika, and cook, stirring constantly, for 3 or 4 minutes or until thickened.

4. Add spinach and artichokes, and stir well to combine. Continue cooking for about 3 minutes or until piping hot.

5. Transfer to a serving bowl, sprinkle vegan Parmesan cheese over top, and serve immediately.

Free Fact

Dark, leafy greens such as spinach, kale, and turnip are excellent sources of calcium and, in most cases, are even better than dairy.

Cheese and Pimento Sandwich

Creamy, tofu-based cream cheese steps in to re-create this favorite sandwich spread flavored with sweet pimentos and briny olives.

1 cup dairy-free cream cheese

2 TB. chopped jarred pimentos

2 TB. chopped green olives

1 tsp. lemon juice

Dash paprika

Pinch salt

4 slices whole-wheat sandwich bread, crusts removed (optional)

Yield: 2 servings
Prep time: 10 minutes
Serving size: 1 sandwich

1. In a medium mixing bowl and with an electric mixer on medium speed, combine cream cheese, pimentos, olives, lemon juice, paprika, and salt until smooth.

2. Spread ½ of mixture on each of 2 bread slices, and top with remaining bread slices. Cut and serve. Cream cheese will keep refrigerated in an airtight container for up to 4 days.

 Milk-Free Morsel

Tofu-based cream cheese spreads are great alternatives to dairy-laden dips for raw veggies and chips.

Grilled Bacon, Cheese, and Tomato Sandwich

A little soy-based cheese goes a long way in this hearty and satisfying sandwich that's a cross between America's two favorites: grilled cheese and the BLT.

Yield: 1 serving

Prep time: 10 minutes

Cook time: 4 minutes

Serving size: 1 sandwich

2 slices whole grain or white sandwich bread

2 tsp. dairy-free margarine

2 slices dairy-free soy-based American or cheddar "cheese"

3 slices bacon, cooked to crisp

1 plum tomato, sliced

Freshly ground black pepper

1. Place bread slices on a cutting board and spread a teaspoon of margarine over each.

2. Heat a nonstick skillet over medium-high heat and place one bread slice, margarine side down, in the skillet. Top with one cheese slice and bacon, cover and reduce heat to low. Cook for 1 minute.

3. Remove the skillet lid and place tomato slices on top of the bacon and add freshly ground pepper. Top with remaining cheese slice, and place the other bread slice on top, margarine side out.

4. Using a spatula, carefully flip over the sandwich and press down lightly. Cover and continue to cook until the bread is golden brown and the cheese has melted, about 3 minutes more.

5. Transfer the sandwich to a cutting board, cut in half, and serve immediately.

Milk-Free Morsel

Look for quick melting rice-based cheeses in your grocery store or health food store if you are avoiding soy products in your diet.

Terrific Tuna and White Bean Panino

Italian flavors of fruity olive oil and oregano highlight this healthy sandwich that's sure to satisfy the hungriest of customers.

1 (6-oz.) can solid white tuna in water, drained

⅔ cup canned cannellini beans, drained and rinsed

2 TB. extra-virgin olive oil

½ tsp. dried oregano

1 tsp. lemon juice

Salt and pepper

4 slices rustic Italian bread, lightly toasted

Yield: 1 serving	
Prep time: 12 minutes	
Serving size: 1 panino	

1. Place tuna in a medium mixing bowl and flake with a fork. Gently stir in cannellini beans.

2. In a small bowl, whisk together extra-virgin olive oil, oregano, lemon juice, salt, and pepper, and pour over tuna and beans. Gently stir to coat.

3. Divide tuna mixture between 2 slices of toasted bread, and top with remaining slices. Press firmly and serve immediately.

Free Fact

Although canned tuna isn't a great source of calcium (fresh tuna has much more), it is rich in B vitamins and is an excellent source of protein and omega-3 fatty acids. Read labels because casein milk protein is sometimes used as an additive in canned tuna.

Hot Turkey Day Panino

Leftovers never tasted so good in this hearty sandwich of turkey, sage-scented stuffing, and sweet cranberry sauce.

Yield: 1 serving
Prep time: 5 minutes
Cook time: 5 minutes
Serving size: 1 panino

2 tsp. mayonnaise

2 slices country-style white bread

4 oz. sliced roasted turkey breast

1 TB. cranberry sauce

2 heaping TB. Corny Cornbread Stuffing (recipe in Chapter 15)

2 tsp. dairy-free margarine

1. Spread 1 teaspoon mayonnaise on each slice of bread. Top 1 slice with turkey, cranberry sauce, and stuffing. Top with remaining slice, and press down firmly.

2. In a medium nonstick skillet over medium heat, melt 1 teaspoon margarine. Place sandwich in the pan, and press down with a metal spatula. Reduce heat to low, cover, and cook for 1 minute.

3. Remove the lid, spread remaining 1 teaspoon margarine on top bread slice, and flip sandwich over. Press again with the spatula, cover, and cook 1 more minute or until filling is hot and bread is lightly browned.

4. Transfer to a serving plate, cut in half, and serve immediately.

 Milk-Free Morsel

Freeze leftover sliced turkey and stuffing in well-wrapped individual servings for quicker defrosting and ready-to-go panino-making or dinner portions. Remember to check for added milk proteins in turkey products, and be sure any sliced deli meats are not cross-contaminated by cheese.

Chapter 7

Outstanding Soups

In This Chapter

- ◆ Quick and "creamy" soups
- ◆ Veggies and grains unite
- ◆ Protein-packed bowls of nourishment

Soup is at the top of many people's list of comfort food, but unfortunately for dairy-free eaters, there's often some dairy lurking in the bowl in the form of butter, milk, cream, or cheese. But thanks to the recipes in this chapter, and some clever substitutes and methods, you can whip up fabulous dairy-free soups in no time.

Obviously, nondairy milks such as soy or almond can step in to mimic the creamy texture we're after. But did you know that many vegetables and grains can do the same? Rice, barley, and starchy root vegetables like potatoes can also create a creamy consistency that's rich and satisfying—and completely dairy free. When blended or puréed, the results can be downright smooth and delicious without any lurking dairy.

Excellent nutrition is on the menu here, too. Hearty soups packed with protein-rich ingredients will keep everyone healthy and fit. Wholesome ingredients abound with every spoonful, and second servings will become the norm.

Creamy Broccoli Soup with "Cheesy" Croutons

Calcium-rich broccoli stars in this smooth and creamy soup featuring a hint of lemon and delicious savory "cheese"-flavored croutons.

Yield: 6 servings
Prep time: 15 minutes
Cook time: 40 minutes
Serving size: 1 cup

1½ lb. broccoli, cut into florets and pieces

1 medium onion, roughly chopped

2 medium Idaho or russet potatoes, peeled and diced

4 cups low-sodium chicken or vegetable broth

1 tsp. lemon juice

½ whole-wheat baguette, cut into 1-in. cubes

Olive oil

¼ tsp. garlic salt

2 TB. vegan Parmesan cheese

1 cup unsweetened soy milk

Salt and pepper

1. Preheat the oven to 350°F.

2. In a large soup pot over medium-high heat, combine broccoli, onion, potatoes, chicken broth, and lemon juice. Bring to a boil, reduce heat to low, and simmer for about 25 minutes or until vegetables are tender.

3. Meanwhile, spread bread cubes in a single layer on a rimmed baking sheet and lightly drizzle with olive oil. Bake for 12 to 15 minutes or until croutons are lightly browned and crispy. Occasionally shake the pan to brown evenly. Remove from the oven.

4. In a large zipper-lock bag, combine garlic salt and vegan Parmesan cheese. Add warm croutons, and shake to coat. Empty croutons into a bowl, and set aside to cool.

5. Add soy milk to the soup pot, and continue cooking for 2 minutes. Remove from heat and begin ladling into a blender up to about ⅔ full. Working in batches, carefully blend, holding a towel firmly over the top, until smooth and transfer to a clean saucepan.

6. Reheat blended soup, and season with salt and pepper. Serve piping hot, topped with croutons. Keep leftover croutons in an airtight container for up to 4 days.

 Milk-Free Morsel

For a somewhat less-smooth result, and to save time and cleanup, you can use an electric handheld immersion blender instead of a blender to finish your soup.

Potato, Leek, and Carrot Soup

Hearty and delicious, this easy soup features the buttery flavor of Yukon gold potatoes and sweet leeks and carrots.

1 TB. dairy-free margarine

1 medium leek, ends trimmed, halved, and thinly sliced

Salt and pepper

4 medium Yukon gold potatoes, peeled and cubed

2 medium carrots, peeled and sliced

4 cups low-sodium chicken or vegetable broth

½ cup soy creamer

Yield: 6 servings	
Prep time: 20 minutes	
Cook time: 30 minutes	
Serving size: 1 cup	

1. In a large soup pot over medium heat, melt margarine. Add leeks, season with salt and pepper, and cook, stirring often, for about 4 minutes or until leeks are soft but not browned.

2. Add potatoes and carrots, and stir to coat. Pour in chicken broth, bring to a boil, reduce heat to low, and simmer for 20 to 25 minutes or until potatoes and carrots are fork-tender.

3. Stir in soy creamer, and cook for 1 more minute.

4. Remove from heat, and using a handheld immersion blender or a potato masher, break up vegetable pieces until soup is somewhat smooth but still a little chunky. Taste for seasoning, and serve immediately.

 Milk-Free Morsel

Although "creamed" soups that contain milk or cream are normally not suited for freezing, soups made with soy or other non-dairy milks freeze very well, so either freeze leftovers or make more to freeze for easy weeknight meals later.

Celery Stalker's Delight

Uniquely aromatic celery root combines with stalk celery to create a satisfying creamed soup that's full of flavor and delicious served hot or cold.

Yield: 6 servings
Prep time: 20 minutes
Cook time: 20 minutes
Serving size: 1 cup

1 TB. dairy-free margarine

1 medium onion, diced

½ bunch celery, trimmed and chopped

2 medium *celeriac* (celery root), peeled and chopped

Salt and pepper

4 cups low-sodium chicken or vegetable broth

⅔ cup unsweetened soy milk

1 TB. finely chopped fresh parsley leaves

1. In a large soup pot over medium heat, melt margarine. Add onion and cook, stirring often, for about 4 minutes or until onion is soft but not browned.

2. Stir in chopped celery and celeriac, season with salt and pepper, and continue to cook, stirring often, for 2 minutes.

3. Pour in broth, bring to a boil, reduce heat to low, and simmer for about 15 minutes or until vegetables are fork-tender.

4. Add soy milk, and continue cooking for 2 minutes. Remove from heat, and begin ladling into a blender up to about ⅔ full. Working in batches, carefully blend holding a towel firmly over the top until smooth and transfer to a clean saucepan.

5. Reheat blended soup, and taste for additional seasoning. Serve piping hot or chill in the refrigerator and serve cold, topped with parsley.

Lactose Lingo

Celeriac, also known as celery root or knob celery, isn't actually the root of the celery plant, but a root vegetable in its own right. Wonderfully fragrant with the taste of celery, celeriac is often used in soups or stews or eaten raw in salads. Its knobby exterior must be ruthlessly removed with a knife.

Creamy Tomato Florentine Soup

Sweet and flavorful *San Marzano* tomatoes highlight this soothing soup with the Florentine touch of nutritious spinach and a hint of fragrant basil.

2 (28-oz.) cans plum tomatoes, preferably San Marzano

2 TB. dairy-free margarine

2 TB. extra-virgin olive oil

1 medium onion, peeled and finely chopped

Salt and pepper

¼ tsp. dried oregano

½ cup chicken or vegetable broth

1 (10-oz.) package frozen chopped spinach, thawed and squeezed dry

½ cup soy creamer

2 TB. chopped fresh basil leaves

Yield: 6 servings
Prep time: 25 minutes
Cook time: 20 minutes
Serving size: about 1 cup

1. Working in batches, process canned tomatoes and their juices in a food processor fitted with a steel blade until smooth. Set aside.

2. Melt together margarine and olive oil in a soup pot over medium heat. Add onion, salt, pepper, and oregano, and cook, stirring often, until softened but not brown, about 4 minutes.

3. Pour in the processed tomatoes and broth, bring the mixture to a low boil over medium heat and allow to simmer for 10 minutes.

4. Stir in spinach and soy creamer and continue to cook for 3 to 5 minutes.

5. To serve, ladle into soup bowls and top each serving with chopped basil leaves.

Lactose Lingo

San Marzano tomatoes are a variety of plum tomatoes from the Naples region of Italy that are considered the best tasting tomatoes for cooking as they have fewer seeds, less acidity, and more sweetness than their Roma tomato counterparts.

Pumpkin-Butternut Bisque

Slightly sweet, silky smooth, and fragrant with the fall spices of ginger, cinnamon, and nutmeg, this soup will hit the spot any time of year.

Yield: 6 servings
Prep time: 15 minutes
Cook time: 20 minutes
Serving size: 1 cup

1 TB. dairy-free margarine

1 medium leek, white part only, sliced

Salt and pepper

1 medium butternut squash, peeled, seeds removed, and diced

1 (15-oz.) can unsweetened pumpkin purée

4 cups low-sodium chicken or vegetable broth

1 TB. light brown sugar, firmly packed

½ tsp. ground ginger

½ tsp. ground cinnamon

Dash ground nutmeg

1 cup almond milk

Sliced almonds

1. In a large soup pot over medium heat, melt margarine. Add leek, season with salt and pepper, and cook, stirring often, for about 4 minutes or until leek is soft but not browned.

2. Add butternut squash, and stir to coat.

3. Add pumpkin purée, chicken broth, brown sugar, ginger, cinnamon, and nutmeg, and stir well to combine. Bring to a boil, reduce heat to low, and simmer for 12 to 15 minutes or until squash is fork-tender.

4. Stir in almond milk, and cook 1 more minute.

5. Remove from heat, and begin ladling into a blender up to about ⅔ full. Working in batches, carefully blend holding a towel firmly over the top until smooth and transfer to a clean saucepan.

6. Taste for seasoning, and serve hot topped with sliced almonds.

Milk-Free Morsel

You can buy butternut squash in packages already peeled and diced to save time and effort. If peeling them yourself, use a sharp knife instead of a peeler for quicker and easier results.

Butter Bean and Kale Soup

Rich, creamy butter beans combine with calcium-rich kale in this hearty soup that's accented with sweet bits of carrot pieces and lots of bold and fragrant garlic.

2 TB. olive oil

1 small onion, diced

1 medium carrot, peeled and diced

Salt and pepper

4 large garlic cloves, minced

4 cups roughly chopped kale leaves, stems removed

4 cups low-sodium chicken or vegetable broth

1 tsp. dried rubbed sage

2 (15-oz.) cans butter beans, drained and rinsed

Yield: 6 servings
Prep time: 25 minutes
Cook time: 25 minutes
Serving size: 1 cup

1. In a large soup pot over medium heat, heat olive oil. Add onion and carrot, season with salt and pepper, and cook, stirring often, for about 3 minutes or until vegetables are soft but not browned.

2. Stir in garlic, and cook 1 more minute. Add kale and stir to coat.

3. Pour in chicken broth and add sage, stir to combine, and bring to a boil. Reduce heat to low, and simmer for about 18 minutes or until kale is tender.

4. Add butter beans, and cook for 3 to 5 minutes or until heated through.

5. Remove from heat, and using a handheld immersion blender, briefly blend just to thicken slightly but leave most beans whole. Taste for seasoning, and serve piping hot.

Free Fact

Of course, butter beans—large white versions of the familiar green lima bean—don't contain any butter. They get their name thanks to their buttery interior texture.

Creamy Southwest Corn Chowder

Hearty and rich with a kick of spicy cayenne and a hint of aromatic cilantro, this soup will please every chunky chowder fan who loves the taste of sweet creamed corn.

Yield: 6 servings	
Prep time: 20 minutes	
Cook time: 25 minutes	
Serving size: 1 cup	

3 strips bacon, diced

1 medium onion, diced

1 medium celery stalk, diced

1 medium red bell pepper, ribs and seeds removed, and diced

Salt

⅛ tsp. cayenne, or more to taste

3 medium Idaho or russet potatoes, peeled and diced

2 (15-oz.) cans corn kernels, drained

4 cups low-sodium chicken or vegetable broth

1 (15-oz.) can cream-style corn

½ cup soy creamer

2 tsp. finely chopped fresh cilantro leaves

1. In a heavy pot over medium heat, fry bacon, stirring often, until crisp. Remove bacon with a slotted spoon, and drain on paper towels.

2. Add onion, celery, red bell pepper, salt, and cayenne to the pot, and cook over medium heat, stirring often, for about 5 minutes or until vegetables are soft but not browned.

3. Add potatoes and corn kernels, and stir well to coat. Pour in chicken broth, and bring to a boil. Reduce heat to low, and simmer for about 15 minutes or until potatoes are fork-tender.

4. Remove from heat, and, using a potato masher, crush some potatoes so soup is somewhat smooth but still chunky.

5. Return to heat, and add cream-style corn, soy creamer, and cilantro. Stir well, and simmer over low heat for 5 more minutes. Taste for seasoning, and serve piping hot sprinkled with bacon bits.

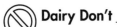 **Dairy Don't**

Canned cream-style corn does not, in most cases, contain any cream or dairy. Gourmet versions, however, might include a splash of milk, so read labels carefully. Homemade creamed corn almost always has added cream, so be sure to ask before eating.

Coconut Curry Soup with Baby Shrimp

Lightly seasoned with just a hint of exotic curry, this easy soup gets its terrific flavor from dairy-free coconut milk and fresh basil.

1 TB. dairy-free margarine

1 medium onion, diced

½ medium green bell pepper, ribs and seeds removed, and diced

½ medium red bell pepper, ribs and seeds removed, and diced

Salt and pepper

1 TB. minced fresh ginger

2 tsp. mild curry powder

4 cups low-sodium chicken or vegetable broth

2 medium red-skinned potatoes, peeled and diced small

1 lb. frozen cooked baby shrimp, thawed

1 (15-oz.) can unsweetened coconut milk

½ cup frozen peas, thawed

3 scallions, trimmed and sliced thin

1 TB. chopped fresh Thai basil leaves

Yield: 6 servings
Prep time: 15 minutes
Cook time: 20 minutes
Serving size: 1 cup

1. In a large soup pot over medium heat, melt margarine. Add onion, green bell pepper, red bell pepper, salt, and pepper, and cook, stirring often, for about 5 minutes or until vegetables are softened but not brown.

2. Add ginger and curry powder, stir well, and cook for 2 more minutes.

3. Pour in chicken broth, add potatoes, and bring to a boil. Reduce heat to low, and simmer for 12 to 15 minutes or until potatoes are fork-tender.

4. Add shrimp, coconut milk, and peas, and simmer for 5 more minutes. Taste for seasoning, and serve piping hot topped with scallions and basil.

Free Fact

Thai basil, a more assertive cousin of the familiar basil used in Italian dishes, can often be hard to find. Look for it in ethnic grocery stores and gourmet food markets.

Cream of Chicken and Rice

Rich, creamy, and full of chicken flavor, this super-easy soup will become a regular part of your delicious dairy-free repertoire.

Yield: 6 servings
Prep time: 15 minutes
Cook time: 15 minutes
Serving size: 1 cup

1 TB. dairy-free margarine

1 small onion, diced

1 medium celery stalk, diced

Salt and pepper

4 cups low-sodium chicken broth

½ cup unsweetened soy milk

1½ cups cooked chicken breast, diced

1½ cups cooked white rice

Dash paprika

1 TB. chopped fresh parsley leaves

1. In a soup pot over medium heat, melt margarine. Add onion and celery, and season with salt and pepper. Cook, stirring often, for about 4 minutes or until vegetables are soft but not browned.

2. Pour in chicken broth and soy milk, stir in ½ of chicken and ½ of rice, stir well, and bring to a boil. Reduce heat to low, and simmer for 5 to 8 minutes.

3. Remove from heat and purée in a blender in batches until smooth and creamy. Transfer to a clean pot.

4. Add remaining chicken and rice, paprika, and additional seasoning if necessary, and cook, stirring occasionally, for about 3 more minutes or until piping hot. Serve immediately topped with parsley.

Milk-Free Morsel

For a heartier meal, save leftover steamed rice from Chinese take-out and add to soups, both homemade and canned.

Chicken and Herb Mushroom Medley

Delicious earthy flavors intermingle in this hearty soup that's thick, rich, and satisfying.

3 TB. olive oil

3 boneless, skinless chicken breasts cut into bite-size pieces

Salt and pepper

1 large leek, trimmed and sliced thin

2 garlic cloves, minced

1 tsp. dried sage leaves

1 tsp. dried thyme

½ tsp. dried marjoram

1 lb. white button mushrooms, wiped clean, trimmed, and halved

6 cups low-sodium chicken broth

1 TB. cornstarch mixed with 2 TB. water

2 TB. chopped fresh parsley leaves

Yield: 6 servings
Prep time: 30 minutes
Cook time: 30 minutes
Serving size: 1½ cups

1. Heat oil in a heavy-bottomed soup pot over medium heat. Add chicken, season with salt and pepper, and cook, stirring often, for 3 to 4 minutes, until no longer pink. Transfer the chicken with a slotted spoon to a clean bowl and set aside.

2. Add the leek to the pot and cook, stirring often, over medium heat for 3 minutes until slightly softened. Add garlic, sage, thyme, and marjoram, and cook 1 minute more.

3. Stir in mushrooms and cook for 2 minutes, stirring occasionally.

4. Pour in chicken broth, stir well, bring to a simmer, and cook for 10 minutes over medium-low heat. Return the chicken to the pot and cook 5 minutes.

5. While stirring the pot, pour in cornstarch mixture and allow the soup to simmer and thicken for 2 to 3 minutes.

6. Taste for the addition of salt and pepper before serving in soup bowls and topping with chopped parsley.

 Milk-Free Morsel

Always wipe mushrooms clean with a damp paper towel rather than washing them in water to prevent sogginess and loss of flavor.

Quick Thick Bean with Bacon Soup

Flavorful bacon highlights this hearty three-bean soup with hints of aromatic thyme and the bold taste of garlic.

Yield: 6 servings
Prep time: 15 minutes
Cook time: 25 minutes
Serving size: 1 cup

¼ lb. bacon or *pancetta*, roughly chopped

2 tsp. olive oil

1 medium onion, diced

2 large garlic cloves, minced

4 cups low-sodium chicken or vegetable broth

½ cup tomato sauce

1 tsp. dried thyme

1 (15-oz.) can red kidney beans

1 (15-oz.) can cannellini beans

1 (15-oz.) can small pink beans

1 tsp. balsamic vinegar

Salt and pepper

1. In a heavy pot over medium heat, fry bacon for about 3 minutes or until almost crisp.

2. Add olive oil and onion, stir well to combine, and cook, stirring occasionally, for about 4 minutes or until onions are soft. Add garlic and cook 2 more minutes.

3. Pour in chicken broth and tomato sauce, add thyme, and bring to a boil, stirring occasionally. Add kidney beans, cannellini beans, and pink beans. Stir well and cook at a low simmer for 10 minutes.

4. Remove from heat, and using a handheld immersion blender or a potato masher, break down beans until mixture is thick but still chunky.

5. Return to a low heat, and while soup is simmering, stir in balsamic vinegar. Season with salt and pepper, and serve immediately.

Lactose Lingo

Pancetta is a type of Italian bacon that's cured, spiced, and dried and often flavored with nutmeg, fennel, and garlic.

Hearty Beef Barley Soup

Nutritious barley combines with tender beef and earthy portobello mushrooms for a soup that's practically a meal in itself.

1 TB. vegetable oil	2 portobello mushrooms, stems and gills removed, and caps roughly chopped
½ lb. stewing beef (such as chuck or round), trimmed of fat and cut into 1-in. dice	1 garlic clove, minced
Salt and pepper	5 cups low-sodium beef broth
1 medium onion, diced	⅔ cup pearl barley
1 medium celery stalk, diced	1 TB. chopped fresh dill
	2 tsp. chopped fresh parsley

Yield: 6 servings	
Prep time: 25 minutes	
Cook time: 80 minutes	
Serving size: 1 cup	

1. In a heavy pot over medium heat, heat vegetable oil. Add beef, season with salt and pepper, and cook, stirring often, for about 8 minutes or until browned. Using a slotted spoon, transfer beef to a bowl and set aside.

2. Add onion and celery to the pot and cook, stirring often for about 5 minutes or until soft. Add mushrooms and garlic, sprinkle with salt, and continue to cook, stirring occasionally, for 3 minutes.

3. Pour in beef broth, and bring to a boil. Reduce heat to low, and return beef to the pot. Cook at a simmer, stirring occasionally, for 40 to 50 minutes or until nearly fork-tender.

4. Stir in barley, dill, and parsley, and continue to cook for about 20 minutes more or until barley grains are soft and beef is tender. If mixture is very thick, add a little water to loosen. Taste for seasoning, and serve piping hot.

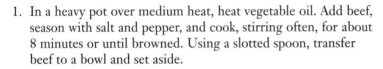

Milk-Free Morsel

To easily remove the gills from a stemmed portobello mushroom cap, scrape them away with the edge of a teaspoon.

Chili Bean Soup

Not too spicy but oh so delicious, this hearty soup flavored with pungent spices, piquant tomatoes, and tasty beef and beans will warm every chili fan to the bone.

Yield: 6 servings
Prep time: 20 minutes
Cook time: 1 hour
Serving size: 1 cup

1 lb. lean ground beef	**1 cup water**
1 large onion, diced	**1 TB. chili powder**
1 large green bell pepper, ribs and seeds removed, and diced	**½ tsp. paprika**
	¼ tsp. ground cumin
Salt and pepper	**Dash cayenne**
1 (28-oz.) can plum tomatoes with juice, roughly chopped	**Pinch sugar**
1 (8-oz.) can tomato sauce	**2 (15-oz.) cans red kidney beans, drained and rinsed**

Free Fact

Texas-style chili, which is the focus of many a chili cook-off, traditionally shuns beans, tomatoes, and other vegetables. Meat and chile peppers are the only accepted main ingredients.

1. In a large heavy pot over medium-high heat, combine beef, onion, and green bell pepper. Season with salt and pepper, and cook, stirring often and breaking up any beef clumps, for about 10 minutes or until vegetables are soft and beef is lightly browned.

2. Add tomatoes with their juice, tomato sauce, water, chili powder, paprika, cumin, cayenne, and sugar. Stir well and bring to a boil.

3. Reduce heat to low, cover, and cook, stirring occasionally, for 40 minutes or until thickened.

4. Remove the cover, stir in kidney beans, and continue to cook for 10 minutes or until piping hot. Taste for seasoning and serve immediately.

Chapter 8

Salads and Salad Dressings

In This Chapter

◆ Innovative salad selections

◆ Dairy-free twists on old favorites

◆ Easy homemade dressings

A healthy diet should include a generous amount of fresh vegetables, and salads are often an easy way to serve up these powerhouses of nutrition. However, salads often contain hidden or not-so-hidden dairy products, whether in the form of sprinkled cheese atop the greens or as milk and cream in the dressings. To help relieve the worry, this chapter provides you with some of the tastiest and most innovative renditions of familiar salads you've ever had, with an ease of preparation that's unmatched.

Salad dressings can be some of the trickiest products to buy with an eye toward dairy free, but making your own has never been easier. From a basic house vinaigrette that can transform itself into a creamy Italian, to the thick and rich favorites of Russian and Green Goddess, you'll be in good stead when its time to dress up! And the added benefit of only fresh ingredients without preservatives will keep you smiling as you whisk your way into the world of salad dressing creation.

Crispy, Crunchy Cabbage Slaw

Refreshingly sweet with a hint of sour, this healthful, fat-free slaw eliminates the need for any milk often added to creamy versions.

Yield: 6 servings
Prep time: 15 minutes
Serving size: ½ cup

1 cup shredded white cabbage

½ cup shredded carrots

½ cup thinly sliced Vidalia or sweet onion

½ cup thinly sliced red or green bell pepper

½ cup thinly sliced kosher dill pickle

½ cup white wine vinegar

⅓ cup water

1½ TB. sugar

Salt and pepper

1. In a large mixing bowl, toss together cabbage, carrots, onion, bell pepper, and dill pickle.

2. In a small bowl, whisk together vinegar, water, sugar, salt, and pepper. Pour dressing over slaw mixture, and toss well to coat.

3. Refrigerate at least 1 hour before serving.

Free Fact _____

The familiar creamy coleslaw didn't appear until the eighteenth century with the invention of mayonnaise. Most slaws were of the pickled variety, such as curtido, from El Salvador, and the spicy kimchi from Korea.

Roasted Baby Potato Salad

Crisp-skinned baby potatoes highlight this dairy-free potato salad that's fragrant with intoxicating fresh rosemary and flavored with robust sun-dried tomatoes and olive oil.

2 lb. baby red or white potatoes, unpeeled and halved

2 TB. olive oil

2 sprigs fresh rosemary

Salt and pepper

1 TB. pine nuts

½ cup chopped sun-dried
tomatoes in oil

Yield: 6 servings
Prep time: 10 minutes
Cook time: 25 minutes
Serving size: ½ cup

1. Preheat the oven to 400°F.

2. Place potatoes in a roasting pan, and drizzle olive oil over top. Add rosemary, salt, and pepper, and toss well to coat.

3. Roast potatoes in the oven for 25 to 30 minutes or until crispy, browned, and fork tender, shaking the pan occasionally to brown evenly. Remove from the oven, drain potatoes on paper towels, and transfer to a medium bowl.

4. While potatoes are still warm, add pine nuts and sun-dried tomatoes in oil, and toss well to coat. Allow to sit at room temperature to cool before serving.

 Milk-Free Morsel

Salads and dressings made with olive oil (without additives and preservatives) thicken when chilled. Always allow them to come to room temperature before tossing and serving.

Carrot, Walnut, and Raisin Salad

Sweet and crunchy with a hint of honey, this terrific salad gets a dab of creaminess from dairy-free soy yogurt.

Yield: 6 servings
Prep time: 30 minutes
Serving size: ½ cup

½ cup raisins

½ cup apple juice

1 (10-oz.) pkg. shredded carrots (about 3 cups)

½ cup chopped walnuts

¼ cup walnut oil

1 TB. honey

2 TB. plain soy yogurt

Salt and pepper

1. In a small bowl, combine raisins and apple juice. Set aside for 20 minutes.

2. In a medium mixing bowl, toss together carrots and walnuts.

3. In a small mixing bowl, combine walnut oil, honey, and soy yogurt.

4. Strain raisins, adding apple juice to the bowl with oil, and adding raisins to carrots.

5. Whisk oil mixture to blend and pour over carrot mixture. Toss well to coat. Season with salt and pepper, and refrigerate for 1 hour before serving.

⊘ Dairy Don't _____

If you're eliminating nuts from a recipe due to allergy concerns, be sure to replace nut oils as well. Try vegetable or olive oils.

Creamy Baby Beet Salad

Delicious little beets get all dressed up in a creamy soy-based dressing with sweet red onion and the crunch of celery.

2 (15-oz.) cans whole baby beets

½ medium red onion, peeled and thinly sliced

1 large celery stalk, trimmed and diced

½ cup soy "sour cream"

¼ cup mayonnaise

¼ cup soy milk

1 tsp. sugar

1 TB. lemon juice

¼ tsp. celery seeds

Salt and pepper

Yield: 6 servings	
Prep time: 25 minutes	
Serving size: ⅔ cup	

1. Drain baby beets, cut in half, and place in a mixing bowl. Add onion and celery and toss lightly to combine.

2. In a small mixing bowl whisk together soy "sour cream," mayonnaise, soy milk, sugar, lemon juice, celery seeds, salt, and pepper until smooth.

3. Pour the dressing mixture over the beet mixture and toss gently. Refrigerate for 1 hour before serving.

Free Fact _____

Beets provide dietary fiber, vitamin C, Iron, Magnesium, and Potassium, and are a very good source of Folate and Manganese.

Picnic Macaroni Salad

Cool and creamy with the tasty crunch of celery and bell peppers, this twist on traditional macaroni salad will have every picnicker clamoring for more.

Yield: 8 servings
Prep time: 15 minutes
Cook time: 10 minutes
Serving size: ½ cup

½ (16-oz.) pkg. elbow macaroni

½ small onion, finely chopped

1 large celery stalk, chopped

½ cup diced green and red bell peppers

1 cup mayonnaise

¼ cup white wine vinegar

2 TB. sugar

2 tsp. yellow mustard

Salt and pepper

¼ cup unsweetened soy milk

Dash paprika

1. Cook macaroni according to package directions. Drain, rinse under cold water, and place in a large mixing bowl. Add onion, celery, and bell peppers, and toss to combine.

2. In a medium mixing bowl, whisk together mayonnaise, vinegar, sugar, mustard, salt, and pepper. Add to macaroni mixture, and stir well. Refrigerate for at least 1 hour.

3. Just before serving, stir in unsweetened soy milk and sprinkle paprika on top.

 Milk-Free Morsel

When substituting soy milk for cow's milk in a recipe, consider using unsweetened soy milk for dishes that are more savory than sweet. Regular soy milk usually has added sugar to counter the natural bitterness of soy.

Primavera Wagon Wheels

Delightful *rotelle* pasta combines with crisp vegetables in this terrific summer salad laced with pungent garlic and the bold taste of sun-dried tomatoes.

½ lb. wagon wheel pasta

2 cups broccoli florets, cooked to crisp-tender

¾ cup peeled and shredded carrots

1 cup canned artichoke hearts, drained and halved

1 cup sugar snap peas, cooked to crisp-tender

¼ cup pine nuts

½ cup sun-dried tomatoes in oil, minced

⅓ cup extra-virgin olive oil

3 TB. lemon juice

1 tsp. grated lemon rind

2 garlic cloves, minced

Salt and pepper

Yield: 8 servings
Prep time: 25 minutes
Cook time: 12 minutes
Serving size: 1 cup

1. Cook wagon wheels according to package directions, drain, and rinse under cold water. Transfer to a large bowl.

2. Stir in broccoli, carrots, artichoke hearts, sugar snap peas, pine nuts, and sun-dried tomatoes.

3. In a small bowl whisk together olive oil, lemon juice, lemon rind, and garlic. Pour over wagon wheel mixture and toss well to coat.

4. Season with salt and pepper and serve lightly chilled or at room temperature.

Lactose Lingo

Rotelle is the Italian name for "little wheels" which gave wagon wheels their American name. In Ohio, where they were first made popular, they are called "choo choo wheels."

Pinto Bean Taco Salad

Bursting with Tex-Mex flavor, this delicious salad, perfect for lunch or picnics, is highlighted by fresh ingredients with a touch of crunch and the salt of corn tortilla chips.

Yield: 4 servings
Prep time: 20 minutes
Serving size: 1 cup

1 Hass avocado, peeled, seed removed, and diced

1 medium tomato, cored, seeds removed, and diced

½ cup finely chopped red onion

½ cup shredded iceberg lettuce

1 (3.8-oz.) can sliced black olives

1 cup canned pinto beans, drained and rinsed

16 corn tortilla chips, broken into pieces

1 TB. chopped green chiles (optional)

½ cup Homemade Thousand Island Dressing (recipe variation later in this chapter)

1. In a large serving bowl, gently stir together avocado, tomato, onion, lettuce, olives, pinto beans, tortilla chips, and chiles (if using).

2. Drizzle Homemade Thousand Island Dressing evenly over top, and toss lightly to coat. Serve immediately.

Milk-Free Morsel

Consider adding diced cooked chicken or turkey to pasta or other salads such as this one to make a main-course salad—and add a good protein boost!

Basic House Italian Dressing

Bold garlic and herbs are featured in this easy and flavorful dressing alternative to commercial brands that may contain milk products and cheese.

1 large garlic clove, peeled and minced

1 tsp. mustard

1 TB. Italian dried herb blend

⅓ cup white wine vinegar

⅔ cup extra-virgin olive oil

Salt and pepper

Yield: 8 servings
Prep time: 10 minutes
Serving size: 2 table-spoons

1. In a medium mixing bowl, whisk together garlic, mustard, herb blend, and vinegar.

2. Slowly add extra-virgin olive oil while whisking until dressing is thick and satiny. Season with salt and pepper. Keep refrigerated for up to 1 week.

Variation: For **Creamy Italian Dressing,** replace extra-virgin olive oil with light olive oil and whisk or beat in ¼ cup soft tofu and a pinch sugar at the end. Season with salt and pepper as necessary.

Dairy Don't

Although most bottled Italian-style dressings are dairy free, watch for those flavored with cheeses such as Parmesan, Romano, and Asiago. If in doubt when dining out, ask for the olive oil and vinegar cruets to create your own vinaigrette.

Green Goddess Dressing

This version of the old favorite gets its thick consistency from rich and creamy avocado without the need for sour cream.

Yield: 6 servings	
Prep time: 12 minutes	
Serving size: 2 tablespoons	

½ Hass avocado, peeled, seed removed, and diced

2 TB. lemon juice

2 TB. mayonnaise

¼ cup olive oil

2 TB. fresh parsley leaves

½ tsp. mustard

½ tsp. sugar

Salt and pepper

1. In a blender, add avocado, lemon juice, mayonnaise, olive oil, parsley leaves, mustard, sugar, salt, and pepper, and purée until smooth.

2. Transfer to an airtight container, and keep refrigerated for up to 3 days.

Free Fact

The original recipe for Green Goddess Dressing is believed to have been created in 1923 at San Francisco's Palace Hotel to honor William Archer's stage play *The Green Goddess.*

Russian Dressing

This simple and tangy dressing is perfect for those who love creamy salad dressing, but without the added milk products found in bottled versions.

1 cup mayonnaise

⅓ cup ketchup

2 tsp. lemon juice

1½ tsp. sugar

Freshly ground black pepper

Yield: 8 servings
Prep time: 5 minutes
Serving size: 2 table-spoons

1. In a small bowl, stir together mayonnaise, ketchup, lemon juice, sugar, and black pepper.

2. Cover and refrigerate for 1 hour before serving. Store in an airtight container for up to 3 days.

Variation: For **Homemade Thousand Island Dressing,** omit sugar and add 1½ tablespoons sweet pickle relish and 1 hard-boiled egg, chopped. Stir well to combine, and store in an airtight container for up to 3 days.

 Free Fact

Russian dressing may have gotten its name from the inclusion of caviar in its earlier recipe versions.

Part 4

What's for Dinner?

How can you cook dinner without a trace of dairy and still satisfy the pickiest of eaters? Are dishes full of creamy richness and delicious "cheesy" flavor a thing of the past? And what about all those classic dairy-laden favorites you once enjoyed?

Here's the best news yet: all your old favorites and comforting classic dinner creations are back on the menu. With a little creativity and some delicious dairy substitutes, you'll be back enjoying all the fabulous dishes you thought were a thing of the past. Creamy sauces and gravies? Rich mashed potatoes? Pizza? They're all here and waiting for you to dive in, so turn the page and get cooking. Your only problem will be what to make first.

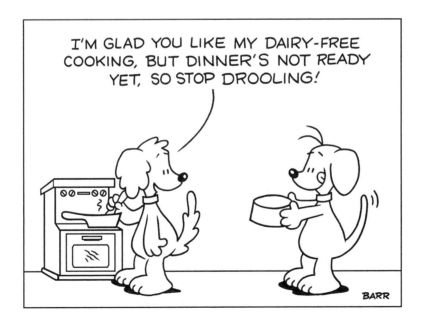

Chapter 9

Meaty Main Dishes

In This Chapter

◆ The meat of the matter

◆ Remarkable richness from dairy-free ingredients

◆ Quick results for fast food

At first, meaty entrées may seem an unlikely venue for dairy, but on closer inspection, many of our favorite dishes are typically prepared and enhanced with a dab of butter here or a splash of cream there. Although far from the main ingredient, sometimes a dairy product provides a particular consistency or flavor we associate with many main dishes, from beef stroganoff to veal scaloppini. Can you really replicate these delicious selections without sacrificing taste and satisfaction?

You bet. Many dairy-free substitutes provide much of the same flavor and texture you're after, while actually reducing the amount of saturated fat. With a little creativity, no traditional dish is off-limits in a dairy-free world.

As an added plus, quick preparations are the name of the game for many of the recipes in this chapter. If you thought dairy-free dinner-making might complicate your life, you'll be happily surprised when you find that simplicity, not to mention taste, reigns.

Pan-Seared Steak with Creamy Shallot Sauce

Dairy-free dining never tasted so good as in this easy and flavorful steak dish, featuring a light cream sauce with hints of sherry and tarragon.

Yield: 2 servings	
Prep time: 15 minutes	
Cook time: 12 minutes	
Serving size: 1 steak	

2 (½-inch thick) top loin (New York strip) steaks

Salt and pepper

2 tsp. olive oil

1 shallot, peeled and finely chopped

½ cup low-sodium beef broth

3 TB. sherry wine vinegar

2 TB. soy creamer

¼ tsp. dried tarragon

1. Season both sides of the steaks with salt and pepper. Heat olive oil in a large nonstick skillet over medium-high heat.

2. Add steaks and cook 4 minutes per side for medium-rare. Transfer to two serving plates.

3. Add chopped shallot to the skillet and cook for 2 minutes over medium heat until lightly browned. Add beef broth and vinegar, increase the heat to high, and cook, stirring often, until reduced by half.

4. Stir in soy creamer and tarragon and continue to cook for 1 minute until slightly thickened. Spoon sauce over the steaks and serve immediately.

Free Fact

Top loin or strip steaks are known by many different names from shell to Delmonico to Kansas City. When called a New York strip, it is always boneless.

Hearty Beef Stroganoff

An unbelievably rich and creamy dairy-free sauce engulfs tender strips of steak over noodles in this comforting entrée.

1 TB. olive oil

1 tsp. dairy-free margarine

1 lb. beef round steak, trimmed and cut into ½-in. strips

Salt and pepper

1 medium onion, diced

1 (10-oz.) pkg. white mushrooms, wiped clean, stemmed, and halved

1 cup tomato sauce

1 cup low-sodium beef broth

½ cup dairy-free sour cream

¼ cup soy creamer

8 oz. egg noodles, cooked according to pkg. directions

Yield: 4 servings	
Prep time: 20 minutes	
Cook time: 90 minutes	
Serving size: about 1 cup	

1. In a large nonstick skillet over medium-high heat, heat olive oil and margarine. Add beef, season with salt and pepper, and cook, stirring occasionally, for about 5 minutes or until lightly browned. Remove beef with a slotted spoon, and set aside.

2. Add onion to the skillet and cook, stirring often, for about 3 minutes or until softened.

3. Add mushrooms to the skillet and cook 2 more minutes.

4. Stir in tomato sauce and beef broth, bring to a boil, add browned beef, and reduce heat to low. Cook, covered, for about 1 hour or until beef is fork-tender. Occasionally stir to prevent sticking.

5. Using a slotted spoon, transfer meat and mushrooms to a warm serving bowl. Add sour cream and soy creamer to the skillet, and whisk to combine. Allow to simmer and thicken for 2 minutes.

6. Taste sauce for seasoning, and pour over beef and mushrooms. Serve with egg noodles.

 Milk-Free Morsel

If egg allergy is a concern, skip the egg noodles and serve this stroganoff over plain white rice.

Marvelous Meatloaf

This terrific entrée gets its flavor from piquant condiments and herbs, and its moistness from eggs and tomato sauce instead of the usual dairy.

Yield: 4 to 6 servings	
Prep time: 12 minutes	
Cook time: 1 hour	
Serving size: 2 slices	

1½ lb. ground beef or beef-veal-pork mixture

2 large eggs

½ cup tomato sauce

1 tsp. spicy brown mustard

2 tsp. Worcestershire sauce

Salt and pepper

⅔ cup seasoned breadcrumbs

1. Preheat the oven to 350°F.

2. In a large mixing bowl, combine beef, eggs, tomato sauce, brown mustard, Worcestershire sauce, salt, pepper, and breadcrumbs.

3. Transfer to a glass or ceramic loaf pan, pat down to remove any air pockets, and form a rectangular loaf. Cover with foil and bake for 1 hour or until an instant-read thermometer inserted in the middle reaches 145°F.

4. Remove from the oven and allow to rest for 10 minutes. Remove foil, pour out any excess accumulated fat, and slice to serve.

🚫 **Dairy Don't**

Watch for commercial seasoned breadcrumbs, particularly Italian flavored, that may contain Parmesan or Romano cheese.

Swedish-Style Meatballs

A rich and creamy dairy-free sauce provides the setting for these tempting nutmeg-scented meatballs that go perfectly with noodles or boiled potatoes.

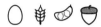

1 lb. ground beef	2 TB. vegetable oil
1 large egg	1 medium onion, chopped
½ cup plain breadcrumbs	1 TB. all-purpose flour
¼ tsp. ground nutmeg	¼ cup soy creamer
Salt and pepper	1 TB. chopped fresh parsley
1 cup plus 2 TB. almond milk	

Yield: 4 servings
Prep time: 15 minutes
Cook time: 30 minutes
Serving size: 6 meatballs

1. In a medium mixing bowl, combine beef, egg, breadcrumbs, nutmeg, salt, pepper, and 2 tablespoons almond milk. Form mixture into 24 meatballs about 1 inch wide, and set on a plate.

2. In a large nonstick skillet over medium-high heat, heat vegetable oil. Add meatballs and brown, swirling the pan to brown evenly, about 8 minutes.

3. Using a slotted spoon, transfer meatballs to a clean bowl. Add onion to the skillet and cook, stirring often, for about 3 minutes or until softened. Sprinkle flour over onions, and cook, stirring, for 1 minute.

4. Whisk in remaining 1 cup almond milk and soy creamer, and bring to a low boil. Allow to simmer on low for 5 minutes or until slightly thickened.

5. Return meatballs to the skillet, and cook in sauce a few more minutes or until piping hot. Serve immediately with parsley on top.

Milk-Free Morsel

This is a terrific dish to serve at children's parties and gatherings where milk allergies may prevail. To be doubly safe, you can substitute the almond milk with rice or soy milk.

Nonna's Italian Meatballs

Simply cooked with the flavor of garlic and marinara sauce, these meatballs are great paired with spaghetti or served on their own.

Yield: 4 servings
Prep time: 12 minutes
Cook time: 25 minutes
Serving size: 3 meatballs

Free Fact

Marinara, originally created in Naples, gets its name from *marinaro,* Italian for "of the sea." In addition to olive oil, tomatoes, garlic, and herbs, early marinara sauces contained seafood from this famous Italian seaport.

1 lb. ground beef	**½ tsp. dried parsley**
1 large egg	**¼ tsp. dried basil**
2 garlic cloves, minced	**Salt and pepper**
½ cup plain breadcrumbs	**1 (26-oz.) jar marinara sauce**
½ tsp. dried oregano	**½ cup water**

1. In a medium mixing bowl, combine ground beef, egg, garlic, breadcrumbs, oregano, parsley, basil, salt, and pepper. Form mixture into 12 meatballs about 2 inches wide, and set on a plate.

2. Pour marinara sauce into a medium saucepan, and use water to swirl out any remaining sauce in the jar. Stir and heat over medium-high heat until bubbly.

3. Gently drop meatballs into sauce one at a time, carefully stirring after each addition. Be sure all meatballs are submerged in sauce.

4. Reduce heat to low, cover, and cook, stirring occasionally, for about 25 minutes or until meatballs are firm and cooked through. Serve immediately with sauce.

Stuffed Peppers with Creamy Tomato Sauce

An old favorite gets a dairy-free makeover in this tangy entrée featuring sweet bell peppers and tender rice, all engulfed in a savory and satisfying sauce.

2 large green bell peppers, halved, cored, and ribs and seeds removed

2 tsp. olive oil

¼ lb. ground beef or veal

1 small onion, minced

Salt and pepper

1 garlic clove, minced

2 cups cooked long-grain white rice

1 tsp. dried parsley

1½ cups tomato sauce

¼ cup rice milk

Dash paprika

Yield: 4 servings
Prep time: 15 minutes
Cook time: 45 minutes
Serving size: ½ stuffed pepper

1. Bring a medium pot of water to a boil over high heat. Drop in bell pepper halves and cook for 2 minutes. Using a slotted spoon, remove peppers and place on paper towels to dry. Place cut side up in a 9×13-inch casserole dish.

2. Preheat the oven to 350°F.

3. In a medium nonstick skillet over medium-high heat, heat olive oil. Add beef, onion, salt, and pepper. Using a fork, break up meat into fine pieces as it cooks.

4. When meat is lightly browned, stir in garlic and cook 1 more minute. Add rice, parsley, and ¼ cup tomato sauce, and stir well to combine.

5. Remove from heat and spoon meat-rice mixture into bell pepper halves, pressing firmly into mounds.

6. Pour remaining 1¼ cups tomato sauce and rice milk into the skillet, and whisk to combine. Cook over low heat for 2 or 3 minutes or until just bubbly, and pour evenly over stuffed peppers.

7. Sprinkle paprika over top of peppers, cover the dish with foil, and bake for about 30 minutes or until peppers are fork-tender and stuffing is piping hot. Serve immediately.

 Milk-Free Morsel

Stuffed peppers freeze particularly well, so double your fun and prepare some extras for another time. Defrost on medium power in the microwave before reheating on high.

Parma-Style Veal Cutlets

Quick and delicious with a hint of sage and a sprinkling of faux Parmesan cheese, these tender cutlets will disappear before you know it.

Yield: 4 servings

Prep time: 12 minutes
Cook time: 8 minutes
Serving size: 2 cutlets

8 (2-oz.) veal cutlets, pounded flat	3 TB. extra-virgin olive oil
Salt and pepper	1 TB. dairy-free margarine
1 tsp. dried sage leaves	1 TB. vegan Parmesan cheese
½ cup all-purpose flour	Lemon wedges

1. Sprinkle veal with salt and pepper.

2. In a shallow dish, combine sage and flour.

3. Heat extra-virgin olive oil and margarine in a large, nonstick skillet over medium-high heat.

4. Coat veal with flour mixture, shake off any excess, and place in hot oil. Cook for about 3 minutes per side or until crispy and browned, and transfer to paper towels to drain.

5. Immediately sprinkle veal with vegan Parmesan cheese, transfer to a warmed serving platter, and serve with lemon wedges on the side.

🚫 Dairy Don't

Restaurant veal cutlets are often dipped in milk instead of egg before breading, so be sure to ask before ordering.

Veal and Mushroom Scaloppini

Here's a favorite restaurant dish made dairy free with the nutty flavor of almonds and the earthy aroma of wild mushrooms.

4 oz. mixed mushrooms (chanterelle, shiitake, *crimini*)

2 TB. olive oil

1 lb. small veal scaloppini pieces, pounded flat

Salt and pepper

1 shallot, minced

¼ cup low-sodium beef broth

½ cup almond milk

1 TB. sliced almonds

Yield: 4 servings
Prep time: 15 minutes
Cook time: 12 minutes
Serving size: 3 pieces

1. Wipe mushrooms clean, remove stems, and slice caps. Set aside.

2. In a large nonstick skillet over medium-high heat, heat olive oil.

3. Season veal with salt and pepper, and place in a single layer in the skillet. Cook for 1 or 2 minutes per side or until lightly browned but not cooked through.

4. Remove veal from the skillet and place on a clean plate. Add shallot and mushrooms to the skillet, season with salt and pepper, and cook, stirring often, for about 5 minutes or until softened.

5. Pour in beef broth and almond milk, bring to a boil, reduce heat to low, and simmer for 1 minute to thicken.

6. Return veal to the pan, submerge in sauce, and cook for 2 minutes or until no longer pink.

7. Transfer veal to serving plates, spoon mushroom sauce over top, and sprinkle with sliced almonds.

Lactose Lingo

Crimini mushrooms, also called "baby bellas" are matured white button mushrooms with a more intense flavor, similar to portobellos, their big brothers.

Pork Chops with Creamy Dill Sauce

Sweet, tender pork chops find a home in a rich and flavorful faux cream sauce with the fragrant hint of dill and the sparkle of paprika.

Yield: 4 servings	
Prep time: 12 minutes	
Cook time: 20 minutes	
Serving size: 2 pork chops	

8 thin-sliced rib or loin pork chops	**½ tsp. paprika**
Salt and pepper	**1 cup low-sodium chicken broth**
Flour	**½ cup dairy-free sour cream**
3 TB. vegetable oil	**¼ cup soy creamer**
1 medium onion, chopped	**1 tsp. chopped fresh dill**

1. Season pork chops with salt and pepper, and coat lightly with flour, shaking off any excess. Set aside.

2. In a large, nonstick skillet over medium-high heat, heat vegetable oil. Add pork chops, and cook about 3 minutes per side or until browned. Remove chops and place on a clean plate.

3. Add onion to the skillet and cook, stirring often, for about 4 minutes or until softened. Add paprika and chicken broth, and bring to a simmer.

4. Return chops to the skillet, cover, and cook on low for 3 minutes or until no longer pink. Transfer to a warm serving platter.

5. Whisk sour cream, soy creamer, and dill into the skillet, and allow to simmer and thicken, whisking often, for 3 or 4 minutes. Taste for additional seasoning, and spoon over pork chops. Serve immediately.

Milk-Free Morsel

If you have extra dill sprigs, finely chop them, combine with softened dairy-free margarine, and freeze the mixture in tablespoon-size discs. Use to flavor steamed vegetables and fish, or spread on bread and top with smoked salmon.

Pork Tenderloin with Honey Mustard Glaze

Lean and luscious, this sliced tenderloin entrée boasts a sweet, tangy glaze and a drizzle of dairy-free richness.

1 (1.5- to 2-lb.) pork tenderloin	¼ cup coarse mustard (with seeds)
Salt and pepper	2 TB. apple juice
1 TB. vegetable oil	¼ cup soy creamer
¼ cup honey	

Yield: 4 servings
Prep time: 10 minutes
Cook time: 35 minutes
Serving size: 3 or 4 thin slices

1. Preheat the oven to 400°F.

2. Season tenderloin with salt and pepper.

3. In a large nonstick skillet over medium-high heat, heat vegetable oil. Add tenderloin, and cook for 4 or 5 minutes or until brown on all sides. Transfer to a medium roasting pan.

4. In a small bowl, stir together honey and mustard, and spoon or brush glaze over pork.

5. Roast tenderloin, occasionally brushing with glaze, until an instant-read thermometer inserted into center reaches 145°F and inside is slightly pink. Transfer tenderloin to a cutting board, and scrape leftover glaze from the roasting pan into the skillet.

6. Add apple juice to the skillet, place over medium-low heat, and scrape up any bits from the browning. Add soy creamer, and stir constantly for 1 minute. Set aside in a warm place.

7. Cut tenderloin on a slight angle into thin slices, and place on a warm serving platter. Drizzle skillet sauce over top, and serve immediately.

Free Fact

Coarse mustard containing seeds add a nice crunch and texture as well as a burst of flavor to coatings and sauces.

Lamb Curry with Yogurt

Soy yogurt steps in nicely for this highly spicy and flavorful Indian entrée that's truly a taste of nirvana.

Yield: 4 servings
Prep time: 2½ hours
Cook time: 1½ hours
Serving size: 1½ cups

1½ lb. boneless leg of lamb, trimmed and cubed

2 cups soy yogurt

1 medium onion, minced

1 jalapeño pepper, cored and minced

1 (1-inch) piece gingerroot, peeled and minced

1 TB. ground coriander

1 tsp. turmeric

½ tsp. ground cumin

½ tsp. ground cinnamon

2 TB. dairy-free margarine

1 large onion, thinly sliced

1 tsp. mustard seeds

Salt and pepper

Cooked basmati rice

1. Spread out lamb cubes in a casserole dish.

2. In a blender combine yogurt, minced onion, jalapeño, gingerroot, coriander, turmeric, cumin, and cinnamon.

3. Pour the yogurt mixture over the lamb, stir to coat, cover, and refrigerate for at least 2 hours.

4. In a large heavy-bottomed pot, melt margarine over medium heat. Add sliced onions and mustard seeds, and cook, stirring often, for about 6 minutes or until softened, but not brown.

5. Add the lamb with the yogurt marinade, stir well to combine, and cook at a simmer, covered, over low heat for about 1½ hours or until tender. Add a little water to prevent sticking if necessary.

6. Season with salt and pepper and serve over rice.

Milk-Free Morsel

When reheating dairy-free sauces that require thinning, add a splash of unsweetened soy or rice milk, rather than water, for a creamier and tastier result.

Classic Shepherd's Pie

A favorite casserole across the pond, kids and adults alike will love the hearty richness of savory meat topped with creamy mashed potatoes and baked to perfection.

1 TB. vegetable oil	½ tsp. dried thyme
1 medium onion, chopped	Dash ground cinnamon
1 medium carrot, peeled and diced	1½ cups low-sodium beef broth
1 lb. ground beef or lamb	1 TB. tomato paste
Salt and pepper	1 batch Super-Simple Mashed Potatoes (recipe in Chapter 14)
1 TB. all-purpose flour	

Yield: 4 servings

Prep time: 15 minutes

Cook time: 40 minutes

Serving size: about 1 cup

1. Preheat the oven to 375°F.

2. In a large skillet over medium-high heat, heat vegetable oil. Add onion and carrot, and cook, stirring often, for about 4 minutes or until softened.

3. Add beef, season with salt and pepper, and cook for 4 or 5 minutes or until no longer pink, using a fork to break up any large clumps. Stir in flour, thyme, and cinnamon, and cook 1 more minute.

4. Add beef broth and tomato paste, stir well to combine, and bring to a simmer. Reduce heat to low and cook, stirring occasionally, for 12 to 15 minutes or until most of liquid has evaporated. Transfer to a 1-quart casserole and spread out evenly.

5. Top meat mixture with mashed potatoes, spreading evenly to cover. Bake for about 25 minutes or until edges are bubbly and potatoes are slightly browned. Remove from the oven and allow to rest 5 minutes before serving.

 Milk-Free Morsel

Make individual shepherd's pies in 6-inch pie tins and freeze for later serving. Defrost and reheat in a conventional oven for 20 minutes or until piping hot.

Chapter 10

Chicken and Turkey Entrées

In This Chapter

♦ Roasting for optimum flavor

♦ Old favorites now dairy free

♦ Turkey dishes you'll gobble up

Whether roasted, fried, or made into terrific one-dish entrées, poultry may well be America's favorite home-cooked main course. You'll see why after you've tasted the delicious dinner selections in this chapter, perfect for any night of the week and all delectably dairy free.

Roasting, which provides super flavor, has long been a favorite cooking method, and thanks to the recipes in this chapter, it will become one of your top choices, too. But old favorites may compete for your applause, because this chapter also shows you how to re-create some of the rich and creamy recipes you may have thought were a thing of the past. Turkey dishes get a makeover here as well, and with the help of some standard dairy-free methods and recipes under your belt, you'll be on your way to cooking all your old favorites, now dairy free.

Soon squawking at the dinner table will become a faint memory when you show them what really great dairy-free cooking can be.

Honey-Roasted Five-Spice Chicken

The exotic spices of Asian cuisine and the golden sweet taste of honey highlight this easy roasted chicken dish full of bold, delicious flavor and moist, succulent tenderness.

Yield: 4 servings
Prep time: 12 minutes
Cook time: 1½ to 2 hours
Serving size: 1 chicken quarter

1 small orange, halved

1 (2½- to 3-lb.) chicken, giblets removed, rinsed, and patted dry

1 TB. *Chinese five-spice powder*

Salt

3 TB. honey

3 TB. dairy-free margarine

1 tsp. grated orange zest

1. Preheat the oven to 350°F.

2. Insert orange halves into chicken cavity, and rub outside of chicken with Chinese five-spice powder. Season with salt, and place chicken breast side down on a wire rack set in a roasting pan.

3. Add about ½ cup water to the pan, and roast chicken for 45 minutes. Turn chicken over on its back, and continue to roast for another 30 minutes.

4. Remove chicken from the oven, and increase the temperature to 450°F.

5. In a small saucepan over medium-low heat, combine honey, margarine, and orange peel, and cook for about 3 minutes or until bubbly.

6. Using a pastry brush, coat chicken with ½ of honey mixture, and return it to the oven for 10 minutes. Repeat with remaining glaze.

7. Continue to roast chicken for 10 to 15 more minutes or until chicken is golden and an instant-read thermometer inserted in thigh reads 175°F.

8. Remove chicken from the oven, and allow to rest for 15 minutes before carving and serving.

Lactose Lingo

Chinese five-spice powder, a popular seasoning for Asian poultry dishes, consists of ground star anise, pepper, fennel, cloves, and cinnamon.

Super-Juicy Roast Chicken

Tangy lemon and flavorful onion help seal in moistness in this delicious, rosemary-scented roasted chicken entrée.

2 lemons, cut into ¼-in. slices	4 chicken quarters (2 thighs with legs and 2 breasts)
4 sprigs fresh rosemary	1 TB. olive oil
1 small onion, thinly sliced into rounds	Salt and pepper

Yield: 4 servings
Prep time: 15 minutes
Cook time: 45 minutes
Serving size: 1 chicken quarter

1. Preheat the oven to 400°F.

2. Arrange lemon slices in a single layer, close together, in the bottom of a roasting pan. Cover with rosemary sprigs.

3. Tuck onion slices under skin of each chicken quarter by carefully loosening skin from meat with your fingertips. Rub each quarter with olive oil, and season with salt and pepper.

4. Place each quarter on top of lemons and rosemary in the roasting pan, and roast in the oven for 40 to 50 minutes or until skin is golden and an instant-read thermometer registers 175°F in thighs and 165°F in breasts.

5. Remove chicken from the oven, and allow to rest for 10 minutes before transferring to a heated serving platter. Top each quarter with some cooked lemon slices, and serve.

Free Fact

Lemons, in addition to providing vitamin C, are a good source of B vitamins, which may be lacking in a dairy-free diet. (Lemons don't provide vitamin B_{12}, however, which is primarily found in animal protein.)

Chicken Tenders with Mushroom Sauce

Tender is definitely the word for these delicious morsels lightly sautéed with a hint of garlic and topped with an earthy mushroom sauce.

Yield: 4 servings
Prep time: 15 minutes
Cook time: 20 minutes
Serving size: 2 or 3 chicken tenders

1 lb. chicken tenderloins, white tendon removed

Salt and pepper

Flour

3 TB. olive oil

1 TB. dairy-free margarine

10 oz. white mushrooms, trimmed and thinly sliced

2 garlic cloves, minced

¼ cup white wine or white grape juice

½ cup low-sodium chicken broth

¼ cup soy creamer

1. Season tenderloins with salt and pepper, and lightly coat with flour, shaking off any excess. Set aside.

2. In a large nonstick skillet over medium heat, heat olive oil and margarine. Add chicken tenders, and lightly brown for about 2 minutes per side. Transfer to a clean plate.

3. Add mushrooms to the pan, and cook, stirring occasionally, for about 6 minutes or until lightly browned. Stir in garlic, and cook 2 more minutes.

4. Increase heat to high, and add white wine. Stir until liquid has evaporated, add chicken broth, and bring to a simmer.

5. Return chicken to the skillet, reduce heat to low, and simmer for about 4 minutes or until cooked through. Transfer chicken to a heated serving platter.

6. Add soy creamer to the skillet, and cook, stirring often, for about 4 minutes or until sauce is bubbly and thickened. Spoon over chicken tenders, and serve immediately.

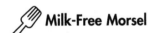

Milk-Free Morsel

To remove the tendon from the tenderloin, hold the thin end firmly while grasping the tendon with a paper towel, and pull from side to side.

Terrific Chicken Cordon Bleu

This classic chicken favorite gets a dairy-free makeover that's just as crispy, delicious, and oozing with rich flavor as the original.

4 boneless, skinless chicken breasts

Salt and pepper

4 thin slices deli-style ham

4 slices diary-free Swiss cheese

¼ cup (½ stick) dairy-free margarine, melted

1½ cups plain breadcrumbs

Yield: 4 servings
Prep time: 20 minutes
Cook time: 1 hour
Serving size: 1 chicken breast

1. Preheat the oven to 400°F. Line a rimmed baking sheet with parchment paper.

2. Slice each chicken breast horizontally to open like a book. Using a meat tenderizer or rolling pin, pound the open breasts to ¼-inch thickness. Sprinkle with salt and pepper.

3. Place ham slices on one side of each breast and top with cheese slices. Close the breasts, tucking in ham and cheese, and secure with toothpicks.

4. Brush the outsides of the breasts with melted margarine and coat with breadcrumbs. Place an inch apart on the prepared baking sheet and bake until crispy and cooked through, about 1 hour.

5. Remove from the oven and allow to rest for 10 minutes. Remove toothpicks before serving.

 Dairy Don't

If buying ham from the deli section of your grocer be sure that the slicers are not also used for cheese which could contaminate the ham with milk proteins.

Crispy Oven-Fried Chicken

This better-for-you oven-fried chicken recipe uses coconut milk for added flavor and versatile corn flakes for a crispy, crunchy coating.

Yield: 4 servings
Prep time: 45 minutes
Cook time: 1 hour
Serving size: 2 drumsticks

8 chicken drumsticks, skins removed

1 (15-oz.) can unsweetened coconut milk

Salt and pepper

2 cups crushed corn flakes

½ cup sweetened flaked coconut

2 TB. dairy-free margarine, melted

1. Preheat the oven to 375°F. Line a rimmed baking sheet with parchment paper.

2. Place drumsticks in a glass or ceramic casserole, stir coconut milk well and pour over chicken. Allow to marinate at least 30 minutes in the refrigerator.

3. In a shallow bowl, combine salt, pepper, crushed corn flakes, and flaked coconut. Dredge each drumstick in corn flake mixture, pressing firmly to adhere, and place on the prepared baking sheet.

4. Drizzle melted margarine over each drumstick, and bake, turning once, for about 1 hour or until chicken is cooked through and crust begins to brown. Remove from the oven and allow to rest for 10 minutes before serving.

⊘ Dairy Don't _____

Read commercial breakfast cereal labels carefully because many contain traces of milk protein. Some may also be processed in manufacturing plants where dairy or other allergy-causing foods may be handled. When in doubt, check with the manufacturer.

Totally Wild Buffalo Wings

The number of alarms is up to you in this homemade version of a spicy delight flavored with paprika and a hint of garlic.

½ cup all-purpose flour

¼ tsp. salt

¼ tsp. paprika

¼ tsp. cayenne pepper, or more to taste

12 chicken wings, rinsed and patted dry

¼ cup (½ stick) dairy-free margarine

¼ cup Louisiana hot sauce

¼ tsp. garlic powder

Freshly ground pepper

Vegetable oil for frying

Yield: 2 servings
Prep time: 1 hour
Cook time: 20 minutes
Serving size: 6 wings

1. In a large mixing bowl combine flour, salt, paprika, and cayenne pepper. Add the chicken wings and toss well to coat.

2. Place the coated wings on a baking sheet and refrigerate for 30 to 45 minutes.

3. In a medium saucepan melt margarine over medium heat. Stir in hot sauce, garlic powder, and ground pepper and set aside in a warm place.

4. Meanwhile heat oil in a deep fryer to 375°F.

5. Carefully drop the wings in the hot oil and fry for 10 to 12 minutes until dark golden and crisp. Immediately transfer the wings to the saucepan and stir to coat well with the hot sauce. Serve immediately.

 Dairy Don't

If you are buying prepared buffalo hot sauce beware that many commercial brands contain dairy in some form.

Quick Pan-Fried Chicken and Gravy

You'll definitely wow them with this version of a Southern favorite that's ready in minutes and served with a delicious white gravy.

Yield: *4 servings*
Prep time: 12 minutes
Cook time: 15 minutes
Serving size: 1 or 2 cutlets

1 lb. thin-sliced chicken breast cutlets

Salt and pepper

¼ cup vegetable oil

1 cup all-purpose flour

1 tsp. paprika

⅔ cup low-sodium chicken broth

⅓ cup soy creamer

1. Season chicken cutlets with salt and pepper, and set aside.

2. In a large, nonstick skillet over medium-high heat, heat vegetable oil.

3. In a shallow bowl, stir together all but 2 tablespoons flour with paprika. Generously dredge cutlets in flour mixture, and add to the skillet. Fry for about 4 minutes per side or until golden brown. Transfer to paper towels to drain, and pour off all but 2 tablespoons remaining oil in the skillet.

4. Reduce heat to medium, and whisk reserved 2 tablespoons flour into the skillet to form a paste.

5. Slowly add chicken broth, whisking constantly to prevent lumps. Add soy creamer, reduce heat to low, and cook, stirring constantly, for 2 more minutes or until thickened.

6. Place cooked cutlets on serving plates. Taste gravy for seasoning, and serve immediately spooned over chicken.

⊘ Dairy Don't _____

Traditional Southern-style pan-fried chicken may often be dipped in buttermilk, and cream gravies are almost always made with dairy, so be sure to ask before trying either when dining out.

Indian Chicken Korma

Mildly seasoned with the fragrant aroma and taste of almonds, this version of a creamy Indian chicken favorite is perfect served over white or brown basmati rice.

½ cup slivered almonds

1 TB. roughly chopped peeled fresh ginger

3 garlic cloves, roughly chopped

⅓ cup almond milk

2 TB. vegetable oil

4 boneless skinless chicken breasts, cut into bite-size pieces

Salt and pepper

1 medium onion, diced

1 cinnamon stick

1 bay leaf

1 tsp. mild curry powder

½ cup low-sodium chicken broth

½ cup plain soy yogurt

Yield: 4 servings
Prep time: 25 minutes
Cook time: 35 minutes
Serving size: about 1 cup

1. In a food processor fitted with a steel blade or in a blender, purée almonds, ginger, garlic, and almond milk until smooth. Set aside.

2. In a large nonstick skillet over medium-high heat, heat vegetable oil. Add chicken, season with salt and pepper, and cook for about 4 minutes or until lightly browned but not cooked through. Using a slotted spoon, transfer chicken to a clean bowl and set aside.

3. Add onion to the skillet, reduce heat to medium, and cook, stirring often, for about 5 minutes or until onion is softened.

4. Stir in cinnamon stick, bay leaf, and curry powder, and continue to cook for 1 more minute.

5. Stir in puréed almond mixture and chicken broth, return chicken and its accumulated juices to the skillet, and bring to a low boil. Cover, reduce heat to low, and cook for about 10 minutes or until chicken is no longer pink inside.

6. Remove the lid, and stir in soy yogurt a little at a time until well blended. Cook, stirring occasionally, for 3 to 5 minutes or until sauce is thickened.

7. Remove and discard cinnamon stick and bay leaf. Taste sauce for seasoning, transfer to a large bowl, and serve.

 Dairy Don't

Many Indian dishes are finished with dollops of cow's milk yogurt mixed in to create a creamy consistency. Ask about the use of ghee (butter) and yogurt when dining out Indian style.

Chicken Stew with Herb Dumplings

Tender vegetables combine with flavor-packed chicken and moist, old-fashioned dumplings in this comfort-food dish that's sure to hit the spot.

Yield: 4 servings
Prep time: 20 minutes
Cook time: 1 hour
Serving size: 2 chicken thighs

2 TB. dairy-free margarine

1 TB. vegetable oil

8 skinless chicken thighs

Salt and pepper

Flour

1 medium onion, chopped

1 medium celery stalk, sliced

2 large carrots, peeled and cut into 1-in. pieces

2 cups low-sodium chicken broth

1 cup water

2 medium red-skinned potatoes, peeled and cubed

½ cup soy creamer

1½ cups all-purpose flour

2 tsp. baking powder

½ tsp. salt

1 TB. finely chopped parsley leaves

½ cup soy milk

1. In a stewing pot over medium heat, heat margarine and vegetable oil.

2. Season chicken with salt and pepper, coat lightly with flour and add to the stew pot. Brown on both sides for about 6 minutes total. Remove and set aside.

3. Add onion and celery to the stew pot, and cook, stirring occasionally, for about 5 minutes or until vegetables are soft but not browned.

4. Add carrots, chicken broth, water, and browned chicken pieces, and bring to a boil. Reduce heat to low, and cook, covered, for 15 minutes. Add potatoes and cook for about 15 more minutes or until all vegetables are fork-tender.

5. Remove the cover, and stir in soy creamer. Continue to simmer.

6. Meanwhile, make dumplings by combining flour, baking powder, and ½ teaspoon salt in a small bowl. Stir in parsley and soy milk just to combine. Drop by spoonfuls onto simmering stew to make 4 dumplings.

7. Cover and cook for 10 to 12 minutes or until a toothpick inserted in center of dumplings comes out dry. Using a large serving spoon, serve directly from the pot into bowls.

 Milk-Free Morsel

Homemade dumplings make a great addition to other stews and soups, and are a terrific alternative to commercial biscuits where dairy may be lurking.

Hail to the Chicken à la King

An old favorite gets a dairy-free makeover in this easy, flavorful chicken and veggies dish in a creamy mock béchamel, perfect for serving over long-grain white rice.

1 TB. dairy-free margarine	½ cup frozen peas, thawed
1 small onion, diced	2 cups diced cooked chicken breast
1 medium celery stalk, diced	
2 medium carrots, peeled and thinly sliced	1 batch Beautiful Béchamel (recipe in Chapter 16)
Salt and pepper	1 tsp. lemon juice

Yield: 4 servings
Prep time: 15 minutes
Cook time: 15 minutes
Serving size: about 1 cup

1. In a nonstick skillet over medium heat, melt margarine. Add onion, celery, and carrots, and season with salt and pepper. Cook, stirring often, for about 6 minutes or until vegetables are softened.

2. Add peas and cook 1 more minute. Set aside.

3. In a large saucepan over low heat, combine chicken with Beautiful Béchamel, and cook, stirring often, for about 8 minutes or until sauce is hot and chicken is heated through.

4. Stir in cooked vegetables and lemon juice, and cook 2 more minutes. Taste for seasoning, and serve immediately.

 Milk-Free Morsel

If you like, you can add leftover vegetables like broccoli florets, asparagus tips, boiled potatoes, or lima beans to your leftover Hail to the Chicken à la King.

Lean, Mean Turkey Loaf

Deliciously moist with a hint of sage and the sweet taste of sautéed onion, this healthful turkey loaf will quickly become a dinnertime favorite.

Yield: 4 servings
Prep time: 15 minutes
Cook time: 1 hour
Serving size: 2 slices

1 TB. olive oil	1 lb. lean ground turkey
1 small onion, finely chopped	1 large egg, beaten
Salt and pepper	2 tsp. mustard
2 tsp. rubbed sage leaves	½ cup breadcrumbs
1 tsp. dried thyme	

1. Preheat the oven to 325°F.

2. In a skillet over medium heat, heat olive oil. Add onion, season with salt and pepper, and cook for about 2 minutes or until onion is soft. Add sage and thyme, and cook 1 more minute. Set aside to cool.

3. In a medium mixing bowl, combine ground turkey, egg, mustard, and breadcrumbs. Add onion mixture, and stir well.

4. Transfer turkey mixture to a glass or ceramic 8×3-inch loaf pan, and pat down to remove any air pockets forming a rectangular loaf. Cover with foil, and bake for 45 to 55 minutes or until an instant-read thermometer inserted in the middle reaches 165°F.

5. Remove from the oven and allow to rest for 10 minutes before slicing and serving.

Milk-Free Morsel

You can make your own fresh breadcrumbs from bread you know is dairy free by tearing it into large pieces and briefly pulsing it in a food processor fitted with a steel blade.

Terrific Turkey Tetrazzini

A classic dish for leftover turkey, this creamy casserole with a crisp faux Parmesan golden crumb topping and flavored with earthy mushrooms will be an instant hit.

1 TB. dairy-free margarine	1 tsp. sherry vinegar
1 TB. olive oil	8 oz. spaghetti, broken in ½ and cooked according to pkg. directions
10 oz. baby bella mushrooms, trimmed and sliced	
Salt and pepper	2 TB. dairy-free margarine, melted
1 garlic clove, minced	⅔ cup plain breadcrumbs
1 batch Beautiful Béchamel (recipe in Chapter 16)	3 TB. vegan Parmesan cheese
2 cups cooked bite-size turkey pieces	1 tsp. dried parsley

Yield: 4 servings
Prep time: 15 minutes
Cook time: 40 to 50 minutes
Serving size: 1½ cups

1. Preheat the oven to 350°F. Lightly coat a 9×13-inch casserole with dairy-free margarine.

2. In a nonstick skillet over medium heat, heat 1 tablespoon margarine and olive oil. Add mushrooms, season with salt and pepper, and cook, stirring occasionally, for 3 or 4 minutes or until lightly golden. Add garlic and cook 1 more minute.

3. In a large saucepan over low heat, heat Beautiful Béchamel until warmed but not boiling. Stir in turkey, sherry vinegar, and cooked mushrooms. Add cooked spaghetti, and toss to coat. Transfer to the prepared casserole.

4. In a small bowl, stir together 2 tablespoons melted margarine, breadcrumbs, vegan Parmesan cheese, and parsley. Sprinkle topping evenly over casserole.

5. Bake for 30 to 40 minutes or until edges are bubbly and crumb topping is golden. Remove from the oven and allow to rest for 10 minutes before serving.

 Milk-Free Morsel

Casseroles like tetrazzini can be made ahead and refrigerated or frozen before baking. If frozen, allow to defrost in the refrigerator before placing in the oven.

Turkey Breast Roll-Ups

In these delicious turkey roll-ups, tender turkey cutlets are stuffed with sweet cornbread and finished with a savory pan gravy.

Yield: 4 servings
Prep time: 30 minutes
Cook time: 30 minutes
Serving size: 1 roll-up

2 Dairy-Free Corn Muffins (recipe in Chapter 5)

1 tsp. dried sage

½ tsp. dried thyme

1 TB. dried cranberries

1 large egg white, beaten

4 turkey breast cutlets, pounded flat

Salt and pepper

1 TB. dairy-free margarine

2 TB. vegetable oil

1 TB. all-purpose flour

1 cup low-sodium turkey or chicken broth

1. Crumble Dairy-Free Corn Muffins in a medium bowl. Add sage, thyme, cranberries, and egg white, and toss gently to combine.

2. Season turkey with salt and pepper. Spread ¼ of cornbread mixture over each cutlet almost to the edge. Carefully roll each stuffed cutlet, beginning at the shortest end, and secure with toothpicks.

3. Preheat the oven to 350°F.

4. In a nonstick skillet over medium heat, heat margarine and vegetable oil. Add roll-ups and lightly brown on all sides for about 2 or 3 minutes, and transfer to a small roasting pan. Reserve pan drippings.

5. Bake roll-ups for about 20 minutes or until turkey is cooked through and stuffing is hot.

6. Meanwhile, make pan gravy by adding flour to drippings in the skillet. Whisk over medium heat until smooth, and slowly pour in turkey broth, whisking to prevent lumps. Reduce heat to low, simmer for about 3 minutes to thicken, and taste for seasoning. Set aside and keep warm.

7. Transfer baked roll-ups to a serving platter, remove the toothpicks, and spoon gravy over top. Serve immediately.

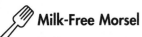

Milk-Free Morsel

To flatten any type of cutlet, place it between 2 pieces of waxed or parchment paper, and gently pound with a mallet or the flat side of a tenderizer to the desired thinness.

Leftover Turkey Picadillo

This super Latin American stew with the flavor of briny olives and capers and the sweetness of calcium-rich almonds and raisins is the perfect foil for too much leftover turkey—and delicious served over rice.

2 TB. olive oil	2 TB. capers, drained
1 medium onion, roughly chopped	½ cup whole blanched almonds
Salt and pepper	1 (28-oz.) can diced tomatoes, with liquid
2 garlic cloves, minced	
2 cups roughly chopped roasted turkey, skin removed	1 bay leaf
	1 tsp. sugar
½ cup pitted green olives, roughly chopped	2 TB. golden raisins

Yield: 4 servings

Prep time: 15 minutes
Cook time: 30 minutes
Serving size: 1 cup

1. In a stew pot over medium heat, heat olive oil. Add onion, season with salt and pepper, and cook, stirring occasionally, for about 4 minutes or until soft but not browned. Add garlic and cook for 1 more minute.

2. Stir in turkey, olives, capers, almonds, tomatoes with their liquid, bay leaf, and sugar, and bring to a simmer. Reduce heat to low, and simmer for 15 minutes.

3. Stir in raisins, and continue simmering for 5 minutes or until stew is thick and raisins are plump. Taste for seasoning, remove bay leaf, and serve immediately.

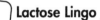

Lactose Lingo

Picadillo is a stew or filling usually made from ground beef, popular in Latin American cuisine and often served with rice and beans.

Fish and Shellfish Dishes

In This Chapter

- ◆ Smooth-sailing shellfish dinners
- ◆ Flavorful fish dishes
- ◆ Delectable dairy-free seafood

In this chapter, you'll find a bounty of meals where fish and shellfish take the starring role. Brimming with healthy nutrients and lean protein, seafood can be one of the smartest things to serve at dinner.

Deep-fried, heavy preparations give way to simple pan-fried versions, while dairy-free sauces and condiments that are surprisingly smooth and creamy help dress up a number of selections from the sea. After you serve some of these fabulous fish entrées, you can rest assured that mutiny will not be a problem.

Easy Fish Fingers

Crisp on the outside and moist and tender on the inside, these tasty fish morsels, free of dairy, will be eaten up faster than you can make them!

Yield: 4 servings
Prep time: 15 minutes
Cook time: 6 minutes
Serving size: 6 pieces

½ cup all-purpose flour

2 large eggs

1 TB. water

Salt and pepper

1½ cups *panko breadcrumbs*

Vegetable oil

1 lb. white, boneless fish fillets, such as cod, cut into 24 strips

Lemon wedges

1 batch Quick Tartar Sauce (recipe in Chapter 16)

1. Set up an assembly line to coat fish: place flour on a plate and set aside. In a shallow bowl, beat eggs with water, salt, and pepper, and set aside. Place breadcrumbs in another shallow bowl and set aside. Finally, place a wire rack over a piece of brown paper at the end of the line.

2. Pour enough vegetable oil into a large skillet to come ¼ inch up the side. Heat oil over medium-high heat until a temperature of 360°F is reached.

3. Dredge fish pieces in flour, shake off any excess, dip in egg mixture, dip in breadcrumbs, and place fish on the rack to set.

4. When oil is hot, carefully place each coated fish finger in the skillet and fry for 2 or 3 minutes per side or until brown and crispy. Work in batches frying 6 to 8 pieces at a time. Allow to drain on paper towels to absorb excess oil.

5. Transfer cooked fish fingers to a warm platter, and serve immediately with lemon wedges and Quick Tartar Sauce.

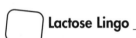

Lactose Lingo

Panko bread-crumbs are a Japanese variety of breadcrumbs, now widely available, that yields a particularly crispy crust when used to coat fried foods.

Golden Crumb-Topped Flounder

Flavored with fruity olive oil and tangy lemon, these quickly broiled fillets feature a crisp crumb topping with a hint of garlic.

4 (6-oz.) flounder fillets	¼ cup whole-wheat bread-crumbs
2 tsp. olive oil	½ tsp. dried parsley
Juice of ½ lemon	¼ tsp. garlic powder
Salt and pepper	

Yield: 4 servings
Prep time: 12 minutes
Cook time: 5 minutes
Serving size: 1 fillet

1. Preheat the oven broiler. Cover a rimmed baking sheet with foil.

2. Place fillets side by side on the foil, drizzle with olive oil and lemon juice, and season with salt and pepper.

3. In a small bowl, stir together breadcrumbs, parsley, and garlic powder, and sprinkle evenly over fillets.

4. Place fillets under the oven broiler, and cook for 4 or 5 minutes or until fish is no longer translucent and breadcrumbs have browned. Turn the baking sheet, if necessary, to brown evenly. Using a metal spatula, transfer fillets to plates, and serve immediately.

 Dairy Don't _____

Some cooks and fishmongers have traditionally soaked fish and even shrimp in milk to remove any "fishy" smell it might have. Be sure to ask about this when eating out or purchasing fresh fish or fresh/frozen shrimp.

Sauced-Up Tilapia

Firm and flavorful tilapia pairs with a creamy béchamel and fragrant fresh dill in this delectable entrée that would be perfect with garden peas and boiled potatoes.

Yield: 4 servings
Prep time: 5 minutes
Cook time: 6 minutes
Serving size: 1 fillet

2 tsp. olive oil	4 (6-oz.) tilapia fillets
1 shallot, minced	Salt and pepper
¼ cup white wine or white grape juice	½ batch Beautiful Béchamel (recipe in Chapter 16), warm
¼ cup water	2 tsp. finely chopped fresh dill

1. In a large nonstick skillet over medium heat, heat olive oil. Add shallot and cook, stirring often, for about 2 minutes or until softened.

2. Add white wine and water, and bring to a simmer. Place tilapia in a single layer in the skillet, and season with salt and pepper.

3. Reduce heat to low, cover, and cook for about 4 minutes or until fillets are firm and no longer translucent.

4. Using a spatula, transfer fillets to serving plates and spoon some warm Beautiful Béchamel over each. Sprinkle with dill, and serve immediately.

Free Fact

Tilapia has very low levels of mercury because it is fast growing and short lived, surviving on a primarily vegetarian diet.

Baked Halibut with Almond Butter

The delicious nutty fragrance of almonds pairs perfectly with softly textured, sweet halibut in this easy baked entrée.

4 (6-oz.) halibut steaks	**Juice of ½ lemon plus 1 TB.**
Salt and pepper	**¼ cup sliced almonds**
2 TB. dairy-free margarine, divided	**½ cup almond milk**
	1 TB. almond butter

Yield: 4 servings

Prep time: 15 minutes

Cook time: 25 minutes

Serving size: 1 halibut steak

1. Preheat the oven to 400°F.

2. Place halibut on a rimmed baking sheet lined with foil. Season with salt and pepper, dot with 1 TB. margarine and sprinkle the juice of ½ lemon over.

3. Bake for 10 minutes, turn over with a spatula, spoon any accumulated juices over the steaks, and continue to bake for 15 minutes until firm and white.

4. Meanwhile in a small saucepan, melt remaining 1 TB. margarine over medium heat and stir in sliced almonds. Cook, stirring often, until lightly toasted.

5. Stir in almond milk, almond butter, and remaining 1 TB. lemon juice and cook for 3 minutes until bubbly. Remove from the heat and season with salt and pepper.

6. To serve, transfer the baked halibut steaks to a warmed platter and spoon the almond mixture over.

Free Fact

Like salmon, halibut is a good source of healthy Omega-3 fatty acids and is also rich in magnesium and many B vitamins including B12.

Quick Poached Salmon

A quick poach in the microwave results in a sweet and succulent salmon entrée delicious hot or cold.

Yield: 2 servings

Prep time: 10 minutes
Cook time: 12 minutes
Serving size: ½ fillet

1 cup water

Juice of ½ lemon

¼ cup apple juice

1 small onion, roughly chopped

1 (2-in.) piece fennel stalk or bulb

1 TB. roughly chopped fennel fronds

1 bay leaf

1 (8-oz.) salmon fillet

½ cup Soy Yogurt Tzatziki (recipe in Chapter 16)

1. In a small saucepan, combine water, lemon juice, apple juice, onion, fennel, fennel fronds, and bay leaf.

2. Bring to a boil over high heat, reduce heat to low, and simmer for 2 minutes. Remove from heat and set aside.

3. Place fillet, skin side down, in a medium-size microwave-safe container. Pour liquid around fillet, cover, and microwave on medium power for 8 to 10 minutes or until salmon is firm but still moist.

4. Remove the lid and let salmon rest in liquid for 2 minutes.

5. To serve, using a spatula, remove salmon from container (skin will come off easily), discard liquid, divide fillet into 2 portions, and serve with Soy Yogurt Tzatziki.

Free Fact

Fennel has long been regarded as a medicinal plant that aids digestion and may even provide strength and courage. Roman gladiators often ate fennel before entering the arena.

Salmon Teriyaki Kebabs

Great for the grill, indoor or out, Asian flavor abounds from a simple marinade of tangy soy sauce, fresh garlic, and bold ginger.

¾ cup soy sauce

¼ cup vegetable oil

2 garlic cloves, smashed

1 (1-in.) piece fresh ginger, sliced

1 TB. firmly packed dark brown sugar

1 (1-lb.) salmon fillet, skin removed and cut into 1-in. cubes

1 medium green bell pepper, ribs and seeds removed, and cut into 1-in. pieces

1 medium red bell pepper, ribs and seeds removed, and cut into 1-in. pieces

Salt and pepper

Yield: 4 servings
Prep time: 20 minutes
Cook time: 10 minutes
Serving size: 1 kebab

1. In a 1-quart casserole dish, combine soy sauce, vegetable oil, garlic, ginger, and brown sugar. Stir well to dissolve sugar.

2. Add salmon cubes, stir, and marinate for 30 minutes, occasionally stirring to distribute flavor.

3. Thread salmon cubes on metal skewers, alternating with green and red bell pepper pieces, divided evenly to make 4 servings. Season with salt and pepper.

4. Heat an indoor or outdoor grill to medium, and brush the grate lightly with oil.

5. Grill kebabs for about 4 minutes per side, turning over halfway through, or until salmon is firm and bell peppers are slightly browned. Transfer to a platter, and serve immediately.

 Dairy Don't

Bottled sauces such as teriyaki and other Asian selections, as well as many soy sauces, contain gluten. If this is a concern for you, be sure to read labels carefully.

Thick and Rich Seafood Gumbo

Oil, not butter, makes a wonderfully flavorful *roux* in this Southern favorite that features the flavors of the sea and a spicy tomato Creole sauce. Serve with plain rice.

Yield: 4 servings	
Prep time: 25 minutes	
Cook time: 35 minutes	
Serving size: about 1 cup	

1 lb. (21 to 30) large shrimp, peeled and deveined

4 oz. bay (baby) scallops

4 oz. swordfish, cut into 1-in. cubes

1 tsp. Creole seasoning blend

¼ cup vegetable oil

¼ cup all-purpose flour

1 medium onion, diced

1 medium green bell pepper, ribs and seeds removed, and diced

1 medium celery stalk, trimmed and diced

Salt and pepper

2 garlic cloves, minced

1 (28-oz.) can plum tomatoes, undrained and roughly chopped

1 cup tomato sauce

½ tsp. dried oregano

1 tsp. sugar

1. In a large bowl, combine shrimp, scallops, and swordfish. Sprinkle with Creole seasoning, and set aside.

2. In a deep, medium microwave-safe glass bowl, whisk together vegetable oil and flour. Microwave on high for 3 minutes. Whisk again, and microwave for 1 more minute or until roux is browned and fragrant.

3. Carefully transfer roux to a large pot, and add onion, green bell pepper, celery, salt, and pepper. Cook over medium heat, stirring often, for about 4 minutes or until vegetables are softened. Add garlic and cook, stirring, for 1 more minute.

4. Stir in plum tomatoes and their liquid, tomato sauce, oregano, and sugar, and bring to a boil. Reduce heat to medium-low, and simmer for 15 minutes, stirring occasionally.

5. Add seafood, stir well, and simmer for 3 or 4 minutes or until just cooked. Remove seafood with a slotted spoon and transfer to a warm serving bowl.

6. Continue to simmer sauce for 5 to 8 minutes or until well thickened. Taste for seasoning, pour over cooked seafood, and serve immediately with rice.

Lactose Lingo

Roux is a mixture of fat and flour used for thickening. French roux is made with flour and butter, while Southern-style roux is typically made with oil. Watch for dishes finished with *beurre manie,* a popular restaurant method of last-minute thickening and flavoring with a butter and flour paste.

Thai Coconut Shrimp

Deliciously creamy with a hint of sweet and a spicy kick, simple shrimp goes Thai in this easy and super-flavorful dish terrific served over jasmine rice or noodles.

2 tsp. vegetable oil

1 small onion, minced

2 garlic cloves, minced

1 TB. finely chopped peeled fresh ginger

½ tsp. turmeric

¼ tsp. ground coriander

1½ cups unsweetened coconut milk

1 tsp. Thai chili sauce or to taste

1 TB. firmly packed light brown sugar

1 TB. ketchup

1 medium red bell pepper, ribs and seeds removed, and cut into thin strips

1 handful baby spinach leaves

1 lb. (31 to 35) medium shrimp, peeled and deveined

¼ cup soy creamer

1 tsp. lime juice

Salt and pepper

Yield: 4 servings
Prep time: 20 minutes
Cook time: 12 minutes
Serving size: about 1 cup

1. In a medium pot over medium-high heat, heat vegetable oil. Add onion and cook, stirring often, for about 2 minutes or until softened. Stir in garlic, ginger, turmeric, and coriander, and cook for 1 more minute.

2. Whisk in coconut milk, Thai chili sauce, brown sugar, and ketchup, and bring to a boil. Reduce heat to low, and simmer for 4 minutes.

3. Increase heat to medium, and add red bell pepper, spinach, and shrimp. Cook, stirring often, for about 5 minutes or until shrimp is pink and firm.

4. Add soy creamer and lime juice, and cook for 1 more minute. Season with salt and pepper, and serve immediately with rice.

Lactose Lingo

Thai chili sauce is a spicy blend of chiles and garlic that's used like Tabasco sauce and added to Thai dishes in small amounts.

Creamy Lemon Shrimp with Rice

The tartness of lemon combines well with the richness of this "cream" sauce and adds piquancy to this easy shrimp and fragrant rice dish.

Yield: 4 servings	
Prep time: 30 minutes	
Cook time: 15 minutes	
Serving size: about 1½ cups	

1 TB. dairy-free margarine

2 TB. olive oil

1 lb. uncooked jumbo shrimp, peeled and deveined

Salt and pepper

1 small onion, minced

¼ cup lemon juice

1 cup fish or vegetable broth

4 TB. dairy-free cream cheese

Cooked *jasmine rice*

1. Melt together margarine and olive oil in a large nonstick skillet over medium heat.

2. Season shrimp with salt and pepper and add to the skillet, stirring frequently until no longer opaque, 3 to 4 minutes. Remove the shrimp with a slotted spoon to a clean bowl and set aside.

3. Add onion to the skillet and cook over medium heat, stirring occasionally, for 4 minutes, until softened but not brown. Add lemon juice and allow to reduce by half.

4. Pour in broth, increase the heat to high and bring to a simmer. Reduce the heat to medium and whisk in cream cheese to make a smooth sauce. Return the shrimp to the skillet, stir well to coat and cook over low heat, stirring occasionally, for 3 minutes more.

5. To serve, spoon shrimp and sauce over cooked rice.

Lactose Lingo

Jasmine rice is a variety of long grain rice similar to basmati, originating in Thailand and highly fragrant with a nutty aroma.

Buttery Potato and Crab Cakes

Buttery-flavored Yukon gold potatoes combine with succulent crabmeat in this delicious recipe flavored with classic Old Bay and fragrant cilantro.

Yield: 4 servings
Prep time: 25 minutes
Cook time: 15 minutes
Serving size: 2 crab cakes

1 large Yukon gold potato, peeled and boiled to fork-tender

8 oz. jumbo lump crabmeat, picked over for shells and cartilage

½ cup mayonnaise

1 large egg white, slightly beaten

1 TB. finely chopped fresh cilantro leaves

1 tsp. *Old Bay Seasoning*

2 cups panko breadcrumbs

Vegetable oil

1 batch Quick Tartar Sauce (recipe in Chapter 16)

1. In a medium mixing bowl, mash potato until smooth. Add crabmeat, mayonnaise, egg white, cilantro, and Old Bay Seasoning, stirring gently to combine.

2. Form mixture into 8 equal-size cakes, and dredge in breadcrumbs. Dredge a second time, and set aside on a clean plate.

3. Pour enough vegetable oil in a large, nonstick skillet to reach ¼ inch up the side. Set over medium-high heat.

4. When oil reaches 360°F or is hot enough to brown a cube of bread, fry crab cakes for 2 or 3 minutes, turning halfway through, or until golden brown. Drain on paper towels and place on a warm platter. Serve with Quick Tartar Sauce.

> **Lactose Lingo** _____
>
> **Old Bay Seasoning** is a classic blend of herbs and spices created in the 1940s specifically for flavoring crab and shrimp. It's named after the ship called the *Old Bay Line* that traversed the Chesapeake Bay from Maryland to Virginia.

Perfect Pasta and Pizza

In This Chapter

◆ Creamy Italian favorites make a return

◆ Nifty noodles and amazing macaroni

◆ Perfect dairy-free pizza

This chapter may well become your favorite after you take your first taste of one of the many dairy-free makeover dishes you thought were gone forever. From a rich and delicious Alfredo sauce to classic macaroni and cheese, they're all here, with some innovative ingredients and flavorful flair.

You'll also find oodles of noodle dishes sure to please. Easy to prepare with simple, dairy-free substitutes, you won't hesitate to take on a new recipe each night. And once the simple Stovetop Mac and "Cheese" is served, you'll be declared the makeover king or queen.

Pizza also makes a return to the menu with a selection of faux-cheese-topped pies and enticing and fresh additions. Before you know it, you'll be whipping up your own pizzas using a multitude of your favorite toppings.

Dairy-Free Pasta Alfredo

Wonderfully creamy and flavorful, with a hint of garlic, this Alfredo sauce, particularly delicious with fresh fettuccine, will delight pasta fans of all ages.

Yield: 4 servings
Prep time: 10 minutes
Cook time: 10 minutes
Serving size: 1½ cups

2 TB. dairy-free margarine

2 cloves garlic, minced

1 TB. all-purpose flour

1 cup unsweetened soy milk

1 cup soy creamer

Dash nutmeg

¼ to ½ cup nutritional yeast flakes, according to taste

Salt and pepper

10 to 12 oz. fresh or dried fettuccine, cooked according to pkg. directions

1. In a large nonstick skillet over medium heat, melt margarine. Add garlic and cook, stirring, for 2 minutes. Do not brown.

2. Whisk in flour to form a paste, and cook for 1 minute. Reduce heat to low, and gradually add soy milk and soy creamer, constantly whisking to prevent lumps. Cook, whisking often, for about 5 minutes or until sauce is slightly thickened.

3. Remove from heat, and whisk in nutmeg, nutritional yeast flakes, salt, and pepper. Serve immediately over cooked fettuccine.

 Milk-Free Morsel

Alfredo sauce is delicious over any type of pasta, so feel free to replace the fettuccine with your favorite pasta. You can even use an egg-free pasta if egg allergy is a concern.

Spaghetti with Garlic and Capers

No need for cheese or any other dairy in this delicious and easy spaghetti dish loaded with garlic flavor and the brightness of little *capers*.

1 lb. spaghetti	Salt and pepper
¼ cup extra virgin olive oil	Dash red pepper flakes
8 garlic cloves, peeled and thinly sliced	3 TB. capers, preferably non-pareil, drained

Yield: 4 servings
Prep time: 10 minutes
Cook time: 15 minutes
Serving size: about 2 cups

1. Begin cooking spaghetti according to package directions.

2. Meanwhile heat olive oil in a large nonstick skillet over medium heat. Add garlic, season with salt, pepper, and red pepper flakes, and cook, stirring often, for 3 minutes until very lightly browned. Remove from heat.

3. When the spaghetti is cooked, drain and add to the skillet along with the capers.

4. Return skillet to heat and cook gently over low heat, using tongs to lift and coat the spaghetti well with the oil mixture until piping hot. Serve immediately.

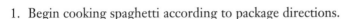

Lactose Lingo

Capers are the salted and pickled buds of the caper plant used frequently in Mediterranean cooking. Non-pareil is the smallest and most desirable size.

Primo Lasagna Primavera

Layers of delectable veggies, firm pasta, and a creamy filling with a hint of basil highlight this favorite dish, enhanced by a flavorful marinara sauce.

Yield: 6 servings
Prep time: 20 minutes
Cook time: 40 minutes
Serving size: 1 (3×4-inch) slice

2 TB. olive oil

1 garlic clove, minced

½ cup shredded carrot

1 small zucchini, ends trimmed, halved, and thinly sliced

1 cup small broccoli florets, cooked to crisp-tender

Salt and pepper

1 (8-oz.) pkg. dairy-free cream cheese

¼ cup soy creamer

1 TB. chopped fresh basil leaves

1 TB. vegan Parmesan cheese

1 (26-oz.) jar marinara sauce

12 lasagna strips, cooked according to pkg. directions

1 cup shredded soy mozzarella

1. In a nonstick skillet over medium heat, heat olive oil. Add garlic and cook, stirring, for 1 minute.

2. Add carrots and zucchini, and continue to cook, stirring often, for about 3 minutes or until vegetables are soft but still firm. Add broccoli and stir well to combine. Season with salt and pepper, remove from heat, cover, and set aside.

3. Preheat the oven to 350°F.

4. In a small mixing bowl, and using an electric mixer on medium speed, beat cream cheese and soy creamer until smooth. Stir in basil and vegan Parmesan cheese, and set aside.

5. Pour ¼ of marinara sauce in a 9×13-inch casserole, and spread evenly with a spatula. Place 3 lasagna strips over sauce, and spread ⅓ of cream cheese mixture evenly over top. Sprinkle with ⅓ of vegetables, and top with a few spoonfuls marinara sauce. Repeat with 2 more layers. Top with remaining lasagna and remaining sauce, and sprinkle mozzarella over top.

6. Bake for 25 to 30 minutes or until edges are bubbly and cheese has melted. Let rest for 10 minutes before slicing and serving.

Free Fact

The term *primavera,* meaning "spring" in Italian, has come to be associated with a pasta dish that features vegetables rather than meat. Its origin is thought to be the celebrated Le Cirque restaurant in New York City.

Rich Rotini Ragu

Hearty and satisfying, this Italian *ragu* of beef flavored with smokey bacon and finished with a creamy dairy-free drizzle clings to its corkscrew pasta with every mouthful.

4 bacon slices, finely chopped	3 TB. tomato paste
2 TB. olive oil	¼ cup soy creamer
1 small onion, minced	Salt and pepper
1 medium carrot, finely chopped	1 lb. rotini pasta, cooked according to package directions
1 medium celery stalk, trimmed and diced	Dairy-free Parmesan cheese (optional)
10 oz. lean ground beef	
1½ cups low-sodium beef broth	

Yield: 4 servings

Prep time: 20 minutes

Cook time: 35 minutes

Serving size: about 2 cups

1. In a large nonstick skillet over medium heat fry bacon in olive oil for 5 minutes, until cooked but not crisp.

2. Add onion, carrot, and celery, and continue cooking for 5 minutes until vegetables are soft.

3. Add ground beef, increase heat to medium-high, and cook until no longer pink, about 8 minutes. Use the back of a fork to break up any lumps of beef.

4. Stir in broth and tomato paste and bring to a low simmer. Reduce the heat to low and cook, stirring often, for about 20 minutes until most of the liquid has gone and mixture is thickened.

5. Stir in soy creamer and season well with salt and pepper. Cook another 5 minutes over low heat, stirring often, until very thick.

6. To serve, spoon the ragu over cooked rotini and sprinkle with Parmesan, if using.

Lactose Lingo

Ragu is the Italian term for a meat-based sauce that is typically served over pasta.

Spinach-Stuffed Shells

Smooth and rich tofu, flavored with Italian herbs and combined with nutritious spinach, replaces the usual ricotta filling in this terrific version of an old favorite.

Yield: 4 servings	
Prep time: 25 minutes	
Cook time: 30 minutes	
Serving size: 2 stuffed shells	

1 (10-oz.) pkg. frozen chopped spinach

1 (15-oz.) pkg. extra-firm tofu

1 TB. vegan Parmesan cheese

¼ tsp. garlic salt

1 tsp. dried oregano

1 tsp. dried basil

Salt and pepper

1 (26-oz.) jar marinara sauce

16 jumbo pasta shells, cooked according to pkg. directions

1 cup shredded soy mozzarella

1. Cook spinach according to package directions, and strain, pressing out any excess water with the back of a spoon. Set aside.

2. Preheat the oven to 375°F.

3. In a food processor fitted with a steel blade, add tofu, spinach, vegan Parmesan cheese, garlic salt, oregano, and basil, and process until smooth. Transfer to a bowl, season with salt and pepper, and set aside.

3. Pour ½ of marinara sauce into a 9×13-inch casserole, and spread evenly.

4. Using a tablespoon, stuff cooked pasta shells with spinach mixture and place side by side, open side up, in the casserole.

5. Evenly spread remaining marinara sauce over shells, cover the casserole with foil, and bake for 20 minutes.

6. Remove the foil, sprinkle mozzarella over top, and bake for 10 more minutes or until cheese has melted and sauce is bubbly. Remove from the oven, and let rest 10 minutes before serving.

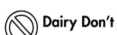

Dairy Don't

Although cheese-stuffed pastas such as stuffed shells and ravioli freeze quite well, dairy-free pasta dishes using tofu as a filling do not. A large amount of water will seep out, and an unappetizing discoloration will result after thawing.

Creamy Noodles Romanoff

Unbelievably rich and creamy with a hint of garlic and a crispy topping flavored with aromatic thyme and marjoram, this noodle dish will become a regular request at dinnertime.

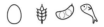

1 (8-oz.) pkg. dairy-free cream cheese

1 cup dairy-free sour cream

½ cup soy creamer

1 TB. dairy-free margarine

1 small onion, minced

Salt and pepper

1 garlic clove, minced

½ tsp. Worcestershire sauce

Dash Tabasco sauce

8 oz. medium-size egg noodles, cooked according to pkg. directions

1 cup panko breadcrumbs

1 tsp. dried thyme

½ tsp. dried marjoram

½ tsp. garlic salt

Yield: 4 servings
Prep time: 20 minutes
Cook time: 30 minutes
Serving size: about 1 cup

1. In a medium mixing bowl, and using an electric mixer on medium speed, beat cream cheese, sour cream, and soy creamer until smooth.

2. Preheat the oven to 350°F.

3. In a nonstick skillet over medium heat, melt margarine. Add onion, season with salt and pepper, and cook, stirring often, for about 3 minutes or until soft but not browned. Add garlic and cook 1 more minute.

4. Transfer onion mixture to cream cheese mixture, add Worcestershire sauce and Tabasco sauce, and stir well to combine. Fold in cooked egg noodles, and transfer to a 1½ quart baking dish.

5. In a small bowl, stir together panko breadcrumbs, thyme, marjoram, and garlic salt. Sprinkle over noodle mixture, and bake for about 25 minutes or until edges begin to bubble and top is slightly golden. Remove from the oven and allow to rest for 10 minutes before serving.

Free Fact

Noodles Romanoff is named after one of the Russian royal families, many of which, like the Stroganoffs, had a particular fondness for rich dishes made with sour cream.

Stovetop Mac and "Cheese"

Who would have thought this traditionally dairy-filled classic could become the richest and creamiest alternative full of delicious "cheesy" flavor? Surprise everyone tonight with their favorite comfort food!

Yield: 4 servings
Prep time: 12 minutes
Cook time: 5 minutes
Serving size: about 1 cup

1 batch "Cheezy" Cream Sauce (recipe in Chapter 16)

8 oz. elbow macaroni, cooked according to pkg. directions

1 cup shredded soy Cheddar cheese

1. In a medium saucepan over low heat, bring "Cheezy" Cream Sauce to a simmer, stirring often.

2. Add macaroni, stir well to combine, and continue cooking over low heat for 2 or 3 minutes or until piping hot.

3. Transfer to a large serving bowl, and sprinkle soy cheddar cheese over top. Serve immediately.

Free Fact

Although urban legend attributes the creation of macaroni and cheese to Thomas Jefferson, the first published recipe for our favorite comfort food dish appeared in *The Experienced English Housekeeper* by Elizabeth Raffald in 1769.

Peanut Sesame Noodles

Sweet, creamy peanut butter highlights this popular Asian dish that features a hint of honey, fragrant sesame oil, and a kick from spicy hot pepper sauce.

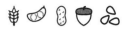

⅔ cup chunky peanut butter

½ cup unsweetened coconut milk

1 TB. rice vinegar

1 TB. honey

1 tsp. soy sauce

1 tsp. toasted sesame oil

Dash hot pepper sauce

8 oz. spaghetti, cooked according to pkg. directions

4 scallions, trimmed and thinly sliced

¼ cup shredded carrots

Yield: 4 servings
Prep time: 12 minutes
Cook time: 5 minutes
Serving size: about 1 cup

1. In a medium saucepan, combine peanut butter, coconut milk, rice vinegar, honey, soy sauce, sesame oil, and hot pepper sauce. Set over medium heat, and whisk for 3 or 4 minutes or until sauce begins to bubble and is heated through.

2. Pour over cooked spaghetti, and toss to coat. Top with scallions and carrots, and serve immediately.

Milk-Free Morsel _____

Rice noodles make for a delicious alternative to spaghetti in Asian dishes for those with wheat/gluten allergies, but be aware that most soy sauces also contain a bit of wheat.

Presto Pizza Dough

It's easier than pie to make a delicious pizza crust from naturally fresh and dairy-free ingredients. The enticing aroma of this yeast dough will lure everyone to the kitchen.

Yield: 1 (15-inch) pizza crust
Prep time: 30 minutes
Cook time: 15 minutes
Serving size: ¼ pie

1 (.25-oz.) pkg. active dry yeast
1 tsp. sugar
1 cup warm water

1 tsp. salt
2 to 2½ cups all-purpose flour
Desired pizza toppings

1. In a medium mixing bowl, stir together yeast, sugar, and water. Set aside to proof (bubble) for 5 minutes.

2. Stir in salt, and add 2 cups flour (or more as necessary) to form a ball.

3. Turn out dough onto a cutting board, and knead for 5 minutes or until dough is smooth. Sprinkle board with flour as needed if dough is sticky. Place in a lightly oiled bowl, and set in a warm place to rise for 20 minutes. (If you're using this dough for another recipe, stop here and proceed with the original recipe's instructions.)

4. Preheat the oven to 425°F.

5. Form dough into a 15-inch-diameter circle, and place on a nonstick baking sheet or pizza stone sprinkled with cornmeal. Add desired toppings, and bake for about 15 minutes or until edges are golden and pizza is cooked through. Let rest for 5 minutes, slice, and serve.

Variation: Use pizza dough to make breadsticks by forming into logs, brushing lightly with olive oil, and sprinkling with coarse salt or dairy-free Parmesan cheese. Bake on a parchment paper–lined baking sheet in a 400°F oven for 10 to 12 minutes.

Milk-Free Morsel

You can make this pizza dough the night before and store it in the refrigerator. It can also be frozen for up to 3 months.

Perfect Pizza Margherita

Fresh, fragrant basil leaves; sweet marinara; and a faux sliced mozzarella help to re-create this classic pizza that's as beautiful to look at as it is delicious to eat.

1 batch unbaked Presto Pizza Dough (recipe earlier in this chapter)

1 cup marinara sauce

8 fresh basil leaves

8 (¼-in.-thick) slices vegan mozzarella cheese

Yield: 4 servings
Prep time: 5 minutes
Cook time: 15 minutes
Serving size: 2 slices

1. Preheat the oven to 425°F.

2. Roll out Presto Pizza Dough to a 15-inch-diameter circle, and place on a nonstick baking sheet or pizza stone sprinkled with cornmeal.

3. Spread marinara sauce evenly over dough almost to the edge. Distribute basil leaves and mozzarella evenly on top.

4. Bake for about 15 minutes or until cheese has melted and crust is cooked through and golden. Remove from the oven, let rest for 5 minutes, cut into 8 slices, and serve.

Free Fact

The pizza Margherita, with its red sauce, green basil, and white mozzarella representing the colors of the Italian flag, was named after Queen Margherita in 1889. She was the wife of King Umberto I, King of Italy.

Chipotle BBQ Chicken Pizza

Smoky chipotle peppers and honey-sweet barbecue sauce highlight this flavorful pizza dotted with tender chicken and baked to perfection.

Yield: 4 servings
Prep time: 15 minutes
Cook time: 15 to 18 minutes
Serving size: 2 slices

1 batch unbaked Presto Pizza Dough (recipe earlier in this chapter)

¾ cup plus 2 TB. barbecue sauce

⅔ cup shredded dairy-free Monterey Jack or cheddar cheese

1 *chipotle pepper* in adobo sauce, diced

1 cup diced cooked chicken breast

1. Preheat the oven to 425°F.

2. Roll out Presto Pizza Dough to a 15-inch-diameter circle, and place on a nonstick baking sheet or pizza stone sprinkled with cornmeal.

3. Spread ¾ cup barbecue sauce evenly over dough almost to the edge. Sprinkle with cheese.

4. In a small bowl, stir together chipotle pepper, chicken, and remaining 2 tablespoons barbecue sauce. Distribute mixture evenly over cheese.

5. Bake for 15 to 18 minutes or until cheese has melted and crust is cooked through and golden. Remove from the oven, let rest for 5 minutes, cut into 8 slices, and serve.

Lactose Lingo

Chipotle peppers are smoked jalapeño peppers, dark in color and almost chocolatelike in flavor. They're available dried, pickled, or canned in adobo sauce, a spicy condiment made from chile peppers that might also contain sesame seeds and peanuts.

Chapter 13

Vegetarian Delights

In This Chapter

◆ *Vegetarian* does not necessarily mean *dairy free*

◆ More than tofu and beans

◆ Delicious international veggie variety

You might suspect that familiar vegetarian entrées are always naturally free of dairy. But unless strictly vegan, milk and its derivatives can show up in any number of places on a meatless menu. From sauces to stir-fries, *vegetarian* does not always equal *dairy-safe*. In this chapter, however, every enticing and hearty recipe is totally dairy free.

Another misconception about vegetarian eating is that, unless you gorge on tofu and beans, you'll never be satiated or nutritionally balanced. As a matter of fact, the hearty dishes in this chapter will not only happily fill you up, but they'll contribute an enormous amount of vitamins and minerals to your diet. For dairy-free eaters, vegetables are actually one of the best sources for finding calcium and even protein. Whether it's grains, lentils, sweet potatoes, or soy, you can't do much better in the healthy eating department.

Plum-Glazed Tofu Stir-Fry

Calcium rich and protein packed, this Asian-style dish flavored with sweet plum sauce and sharp ginger is a delicious departure from meaty entrées.

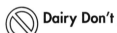

> *Yield: 4 servings*
>
> **Prep time:** 20 minutes
> **Cook time:** 15 minutes
> **Serving size:** about 1 cup

1 lb. extra-firm tofu, halved vertically and cut into 16 slices

Salt and pepper

1 TB. vegetable oil

½ red bell pepper, ribs and seeds removed, and sliced

1 bunch scallions, trimmed and cut into 2-in. pieces

1 cup canned Asian baby corn, drained

½ cup sliced water chestnuts, drained

½ cup vegetable broth

½ cup plum jam

1 TB. finely chopped peeled fresh ginger

1 TB. lemon juice

1 tsp. soy sauce

Dairy Don't

Commercially pre-pared Asian sauces and condiments can be convenient, but when these products are imported, such as the ones we often see at Asian markets, labeling can be a problem because strict adherence to ingredient facts may not hold. If in doubt, err on the side of caution and purchase similar products with clearer labeling.

1. Press tofu slices between paper towels to remove excess liquid. Season with salt and pepper.

2. In a large nonstick skillet or wok, heat vegetable oil over high heat. Carefully place tofu slices in the skillet, and brown lightly 1 or 2 minutes per side. Remove with a spatula and set aside.

3. Add red bell pepper and scallions to the skillet, and cook, stirring constantly, for about 2 minutes or until somewhat softened. Add baby corn and water chestnuts, and cook for 1 more minute.

4. Reduce heat to low, pour in vegetable broth, return tofu slices to the skillet, cover, and cook for 2 minutes.

5. Meanwhile, in a small bowl, stir together plum jam, ginger, lemon juice, and soy sauce.

6. Remove the skillet lid, add plum sauce, and gently stir tofu and vegetables to coat. Cook 1 or 2 more minutes or until thick and bubbly. Transfer to a bowl, and serve immediately with rice, if desired.

Oven-Baked Tempeh with Sweet Potatoes

Roasting sweet potatoes brings out their finest flavor, while aromatic spices and savory soy enhance this vegetarian *tempeh* entrée.

Yield: *4 servings*	
Prep time: 20 minutes	
Cook time: 40 minutes	
Serving size: about 1 cup	

¼ cup soy sauce

1 TB. rice vinegar

1 tsp. sugar

¼ tsp. garlic powder

¼ tsp. onion powder

2 tsp. toasted sesame oil

8 oz. tempeh, cut into 1-in. cubes

2 medium sweet potatoes, peeled and cubed

2 TB. vegetable oil

Salt and pepper

Dash ground ginger

Dash ground cinnamon

1. In a shallow dish, combine soy sauce, rice vinegar, sugar, garlic powder, onion powder, and sesame oil. Add cubed tempeh, stir to coat, and set aside to marinate for 15 minutes.

2. Preheat the oven to 350°F.

3. In a large roasting pan, combine cubed sweet potatoes, 1 tablespoon vegetable oil, salt, pepper, ginger, and cinnamon. Toss well to coat.

4. Heat remaining 1 tablespoon vegetable oil in a medium nonstick skillet over medium-high heat. Add tempeh pieces, and fry for about 2 minutes per side or until browned. Remove from heat, add to sweet potatoes in the roasting pan, and toss to combine.

5. Roast in the oven for 25 to 30 minutes or until sweet potatoes are fork-tender and lightly browned. Taste for additional seasoning, and serve.

Lactose Lingo

Tempeh is a fermented soybean product popular in Indonesia and used frequently in vegetarian cooking. Unlike tofu, the beans stay whole, forming a cake that contains higher levels of protein, fiber, nutrients, and flavor.

Kasha Varnishkes with Sweet Onions and Carrots

Yield: 2 servings
Prep time: 10 minutes
Cook time: 25 minutes
Serving size: 2 cups

Kasha's nutty flavor pairs well with sweet caramelized onion and carrots in this hearty dish featuring bowtie pasta.

¾ cup medium-grain kasha

1 large egg, slightly beaten

1 TB. vegetable oil

2 tsp. dairy-free margarine

1 medium onion, halved and thinly sliced

1 cup shredded carrots

Salt and pepper

1½ cups low-sodium vegetable broth

1½ cups bowtie pasta

1. In a medium mixing bowl, add kasha and stir in beaten egg, being sure to coat each grain.

2. In a large nonstick skillet over medium-high heat, heat vegetable oil and margarine. Add onion and carrots, season with salt and pepper, and cook, stirring often, for about 5 minutes or until vegetables are softened and slightly browned.

3. Add kasha to the skillet and, using the back of a fork, break up any clumps. Cook for 3 or 4 minutes, stirring constantly, until egg has dried and kasha begins to toast.

4. Pour in vegetable broth, bring to a boil, reduce heat to low, cover, and cook for 10 to 15 minutes or until kasha is tender.

5. Cook bowtie pasta according to package directions and drain well.

6. Add cooked bowtie pasta, stir to combine well, and cook for 3 or 4 more minutes or until piping hot. Taste for seasoning, and serve immediately.

🚫 **Dairy Don't**

Although the religious term Pareve indicates that a food is generally milk free, according to Jewish dietary rules, the Pareve label is allowable even if traces of milk derivatives exist. Be sure to read labels carefully.

Baked Rigatoni with Tofu

Tofu provides the protein while mimicking the texture of cheese in this delicious cousin to baked ziti, enticingly fragrant with fresh basil.

1 (26-oz.) jar marinara or spaghetti sauce

1 lb. rigatoni pasta, cooked according to package directions

½ lb. firm tofu, drained, and cut into medium cubes

2 TB. fresh basil leaves, cut into julienne

Freshly ground black pepper

1 cup shredded dairy-free mozzarella cheese

Yield: 6 servings
Prep time: 20 minutes
Cook time: 30 minutes
Serving size: about 1½ cups

1. Preheat the oven to 350°F.

2. Spread ⅓ of the sauce in the bottom of a 9×13-inch casserole. Spoon half the cooked rigatoni on top and sprinkle with half the tofu and basil leaves, finishing with a grinding of black pepper.

3. Spread half the remaining sauce on top and add the remaining rigatoni, tofu, and basil as above. Finish with the remaining sauce, some black pepper, and the mozzarella cheese.

4. Bake for 30 minutes until the edges are bubbly and the cheese has melted. Remove from the oven and allow to rest for 10 minutes before serving.

 Milk-Free Morsel

To cut basil leaves into julienne strips, place 3 or 4 stemmed leaves on top of each other and roll up like a cigar. Cut ⅛-inch thick slices from end to end, then toss lightly to release the strips of basil.

Vegetarian Moussaka

This Greek favorite with a hint of spice and a burst of fresh herbs gets a meatless makeover with the addition of savory lentils and a creamy, kicked-up dairy-free béchamel sauce.

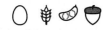

Yield: 4 servings
Prep time: 15 minutes
Cook time: 60 minutes
Serving size: about 1 cup

1 large eggplant, peeled and cut into ½-in. slices

Salt and pepper

¼ cup olive oil, or more for frying

1 (15-oz.) can cooked brown lentils, drained and rinsed

½ cup tomato sauce

1½ TB. chopped fresh parsley leaves

1 tsp. chopped fresh thyme leaves

1½ cups Beautiful Béchamel Sauce (recipe in Chapter 16)

1 large egg, beaten

2 TB. vegan Parmesan cheese

Pinch paprika

1. Preheat the oven to 350°F.

2. Season eggplant slices with salt and pepper.

3. In a large nonstick skillet over medium-high heat, heat olive oil. Add eggplant, and fry for 3 minutes per side or until lightly browned and softened. Add more oil to the skillet, if necessary. Drain eggplant on a paper towel and set aside.

4. In a medium saucepan over medium heat, combine lentils, tomato sauce, salt, pepper, parsley, and thyme. Cook, stirring often, for 5 or 6 minutes or until piping hot. Remove from heat.

5. Place ½ of eggplant slices in the bottom of a 1-quart casserole dish. Spread lentil mixture evenly over, and top with remaining eggplant slices.

6. In a medium saucepan over low heat, whisk together Beautiful Béchamel Sauce, egg, and vegan Parmesan cheese until mixture begins to bubble. Pour over top of casserole, and spread evenly. Sprinkle with paprika, and bake 30 to 35 minutes or until top is puffed and edges are bubbly. Serve immediately.

Milk-Free Morsel

Casseroles such as moussaka lend themselves to make-ahead preparation and even freezing. Consider creating individual servings in small casserole dishes or doubling the recipe to freeze part of it for later use.

Cornbread Chili Bean Casserole

Spicy vegetarian chili is topped with a cover of sweet cornbread in this one-dish meal full of flavor and packed with protein.

Yield: *4 servings*		
Prep time: 10 minutes		
Cook time: 40 minutes		
Serving size: about 1 cup		

1 TB. vegetable oil	2 cups canned pinto or kidney beans, drained and rinsed
1 medium onion, chopped	
1 medium green bell pepper, ribs and seeds removed, and diced	¾ cup soy milk
	1 tsp. cider vinegar
Salt and pepper	1 cup all-purpose flour
1 TB. chili powder	⅔ cup stone-ground yellow cornmeal
1 tsp. ground cumin	
1 tsp. paprika	1 TB. sugar
¼ tsp. cayenne	1½ tsp. baking powder
1 cup water	½ tsp. salt
1 cup canned diced tomatoes, undrained	1 large egg, beaten

1. In a large nonstick skillet over medium-high heat, heat vegetable oil. Add onion and bell pepper, season with salt and pepper, and cook, stirring often, for 4 minutes or until softened.

2. Stir in chili powder, cumin, paprika, and cayenne, and cook for 1 more minute. Add water and tomatoes with their juice, and bring to a boil.

3. Stir in pinto beans, reduce heat to low, and cook for 10 to 12 minutes or until thick and piping hot. Transfer to a 1-quart casserole.

4. Preheat the oven to 350°F.

5. In a small bowl, stir together soy milk and cider vinegar. Set aside for 5 minutes.

6. Meanwhile, in a medium mixing bowl, whisk together flour, cornmeal, sugar, baking powder, and ½ teaspoon salt.

7. Add beaten egg to soy milk mixture, and combine with flour mixture, stirring just to blend. Drop spoonfuls of mixture on top of chili beans without spreading out.

8. Bake for 22 to 25 minutes or until casserole is bubbly and cornmeal topping is puffed and lightly browned. Allow to rest for 5 minutes before serving.

 Milk-Free Morsel

A great substitute for buttermilk is plain milk mixed with a little vinegar. Using soy milk or another dairy-free milk provides the same results.

Vegetable Curry with Creamy Coconut Rice

Exotic Indian flavor highlights this medley of nutritious vegetables served with a creamy, tropical-flavored coconut rice.

1 TB. vegetable oil

½ medium onion, roughly chopped

½ medium red bell pepper, ribs and seeds removed, and diced

Salt and pepper

1 TB. minced peeled fresh ginger

2 garlic cloves, minced

½ small jalapeño pepper, seeds removed, and minced

1 TB. curry powder

½ tsp. ground turmeric

¼ tsp. ground coriander

2 cups vegetable broth

½ cup tomato sauce

¼ cup dried red lentils

2 red potatoes, peeled and cubed

1 cup cauliflower florets

½ cup sliced carrots

¼ cup frozen peas

1 cup white basmati rice

1 cup water

1 cup unsweetened coconut milk

Pinch salt

2 TB. cream of coconut

Yield: 4 servings
Prep time: 20 minutes
Cook time: 30 minutes
Serving size: about 2 cups

1. In a large pot over medium-high heat, heat vegetable oil. Add onion, red bell pepper, salt, and pepper, and cook, stirring often, for about 3 minutes or until softened.

2. Add ginger, garlic, and jalapeño, and cook, stirring, for 1 more minute. Add curry powder, turmeric, and coriander, and stir well to coat vegetables.

3. Add vegetable broth and tomato sauce, and bring to a boil. Add lentils, potatoes, cauliflower, carrots, and peas. Reduce heat to low, cover, and simmer for 12 to 15 minutes or until vegetables are tender and lentils are soft.

 Milk-Free Morsel

The addition of a small amount of red lentils to curries and stews helps thicken the sauce without the need for any butter-laden roux or cream.

4. Meanwhile, combine rice, water, coconut milk, and pinch salt in a medium saucepan and bring to a boil over high heat. Reduce heat to low, cover, and cook for about 12 minutes or until rice is tender and liquid is absorbed. Stir in cream of coconut, and set aside, covered, to keep warm.

5. When vegetables are tender, remove them with a slotted spoon to a serving bowl. Taste sauce for seasoning, and adjust if necessary. Simmer for 1 or 2 minutes to reduce slightly, pour over vegetables, and serve with coconut rice.

Fabulous Falafel Patties

Spiced up chickpeas that are full of flavor are the basis of this tasty meatless and dairy-free Middle Eastern delight.

2 (15-oz.) cans chickpeas, drained and rinsed	½ tsp. salt
1 small onion, finely chopped	½ tsp. ground cumin
¼ cup finely chopped fresh parsley leaves	¼ tsp. ground coriander
	Dash cayenne pepper
¼ cup toasted wheat germ	1 cup all-purpose flour
1 large egg white	Vegetable oil for frying
1 TB. lemon juice	Soy Yogurt Tzaziki (recipe in Chapter 16; optional)
¾ tsp. baking soda	

Yield: 4 servings
Prep time: 30 minutes
Cook time: 15 minutes
Serving size: 4 patties

1. In the bowl of a food processor fitted with a steel blade combine chickpeas (reserving ½ cup for later use), and the onion, parsley, wheat germ, egg white, lemon juice, baking soda, salt, cumin, coriander, and cayenne pepper.

2. Purée about 1 minute until smooth. Add remaining chickpeas and pulse a few times so there are small pieces of chickpea visible.

3. Form the mixture into 16 patties and place on a baking sheet lined with parchment. Refrigerate for 25 minutes.

4. Place flour in a shallow bowl. Heat enough oil in a large nonstick skillet over medium-high heat to come ¼ inch up the side.

5. When oil is hot, dip the patties in the flour on both sides, lightly patting away any excess flour, and fry in batches in the skillet for 3 or 4 minutes per side until golden brown.

6. Transfer fried patties to a paper towel to drain. Serve hot with Soy Yogurt Tzaziki sauce, if desired.

 Dairy Don't _____

If ordering a plate of falafel or a falafel sandwich when dining out be sure to ask that any yogurt sauce not be included for those who are allergic to milk protein.

Roasted Vegetable Burritos

A delicious take on a Mexican favorite, this healthful, dairy-free version features the aromatic flavor of fresh basil and a hint of Parmesan.

Yield: 2 servings

Prep time: 15 minutes
Cook time: 20 minutes
Serving size: 2 burritos

1 small eggplant, peeled and cut into ½-in. dice

1 medium zucchini, trimmed and cut into ½-in. circles

1 medium red bell pepper, ribs and seeds removed, and sliced

1 small red onion, halved and thinly sliced

2 TB. olive oil

Salt and pepper

4 burrito-size flour tortillas, warmed

1 TB. chopped fresh basil

1 TB. vegan Parmesan cheese

1. Preheat the oven to 375°F.

2. In a roasting pan, combine eggplant, zucchini, red bell pepper, onion, olive oil, salt, and pepper, and toss well to coat.

3. Roast vegetables, shaking the pan occasionally, for 20 minutes or until lightly browned and fork-tender.

4. Divide vegetables among 4 tortillas, and arrange in the middle of each tortilla. Sprinkle basil and Parmesan over each, fold up burrito style, and serve immediately.

Milk-Free Morsel

Make burritos ahead of time, enclose in a zipper-lock bag, and take along for lunch or snacking. When ready to eat, a quick minute in the microwave while still in the bag is all you need.

Chapter **14**

Vegetables on the Side

In This Chapter

- ◆ Spud dishes galore!
- ◆ Get your fill of delicious, nutritious greens
- ◆ Sauce it up, completely dairy free

Potato side dishes in a multitude of forms are probably the most popular American sides we order when eating out. But dairy products can lurk in even a simple baked potato. Butter, sour cream, milk, and cheese are common partners for spuds, so must we give up our favorite side to be dairy safe? Certainly not! In this chapter, you find all your favorite potato recipes made completely dairy free without sacrificing flavor, taste, or consistency.

As much as we love our spuds, numerous other nutritious and delicious vegetables are available to enjoy. From broccoli to spinach to asparagus, nutrient-packed veggies are a smart choice, especially when seeking B vitamins and calcium. You'll find terrific preparations for many favorites, full of flavor and far from bland. Before long, you and your family won't feel at all deprived as you enjoy every last morsel of these stellar sides that simply ooze with flavor and pop with culinary style.

Healthy Homemade Fries

If concerns about hidden dairy or cross-contamination have kept you from enjoying French fries, these crispy and flavorful oven fries will definitely fit the bill.

Yield: 4 servings
Prep time: 10 minutes
Cook time: 40 minutes
Serving size: 8 fries

4 medium Idaho or russet potatoes

2 TB. vegetable oil

Salt and pepper

1. Preheat the oven to 400°F.

2. Peel potatoes and cut each in half lengthwise. Cut each half into 4 wedges and place in a bowl of cold water.

3. Brush a rimmed baking sheet with 1 TB. of oil. Drain the potatoes and pat dry with paper towels.

4. Lay the potato wedges on the baking sheet in a single layer and brush each with the remaining 1 TB. oil. Sprinkle with salt and pepper.

5. Bake for about 20 minutes per side, or until crisp and golden. Serve immediately.

🚫 **Dairy Don't** _____

Some fast food restaurants add flavoring to their fries which may contain milk protein. Similarly, cross-contamination is a possibility through the sharing of kitchen utensils and fryers, so always be cautious when ordering out.

Twice-Baked Stuffed Potatoes

Crispy potato skins hold a surprisingly creamy, buttery-flavored filling topped with aromatic fresh chopped chives and a dash of paprika.

4 medium Idaho or russet potatoes, baked

1 tsp. vegetable oil

2 TB. dairy-free margarine

⅓ cup soy creamer

1 tsp. mustard

Salt and pepper

Dash paprika

1 TB. chopped fresh chives

Yield: 4 servings
Prep time: 10 minutes
Cook time: 25 minutes
Serving size: 1 potato

1. Preheat the oven to 400°F.

2. While potatoes are still warm, use a sharp paring knife to cut out a long, narrow opening on the top of each potato and discard. Scoop out all but ¼ inch of pulp from each potato, and place it in a medium mixing bowl.

3. Lightly brush potato skins with vegetable oil, place on a baking sheet, and bake for 5 to 8 minutes or until crispy.

4. Meanwhile, add margarine, soy creamer, mustard, salt, and pepper to potato pulp and beat with an electric mixer on medium speed for 1 or 2 minutes or until smooth and creamy.

5. Fill each crisped potato skin with stuffing, sprinkle with paprika, and return to the oven for 12 to 15 minutes or until piping hot. Sprinkle tops with chopped fresh chives just before serving.

Milk-Free Morsel

Keep fresh chives fresh by wrapping them in a damp paper towel and placing them in an open zipper-lock bag in your refrigerator's vegetable bin.

Delicious Potatoes No Gratin

This milk- and cheese-free "gratin" of layered potatoes gets its buttery flavor from Yukon gold potatoes and its savory delight from chicken broth and fresh thyme.

Yield: 4 servings
Prep time: 20 minutes
Cook time: 45 minutes
Serving size: about ⅔ cup

2 lb. Yukon gold potatoes, peeled and sliced thin

Salt and pepper

2 tsp. chopped fresh thyme leaves

2 cups low-sodium chicken broth, hot

1. Preheat the oven to 400°F. Lightly coat the bottom and sides of a 2-quart casserole dish with olive oil.

2. In a large bowl, toss together potato slices, salt, pepper, and fresh thyme. Transfer to the prepared casserole dish, and spread out evenly.

3. Pour chicken broth over potatoes, cover with foil, and bake for 25 minutes. Remove the foil, and continue to bake, occasionally basting potatoes with liquid, for 20 more minutes or until potatoes are fork-tender and have begun to brown.

4. Remove from the oven and allow to rest 5 minutes before serving.

Free Fact

Yukon gold potatoes, now a staple in supermarket produce sections, were developed in Canada as recently as the early 1980s. They are now universally loved for their golden, buttery-tasting flesh.

Super-Simple Mashed Potatoes

Soy creamer and dairy-free margarine step in for an amazingly rich and delicious version of quick mashed potatoes sure to become a staple side at dinner time.

2 lb. Idaho, russet, or Yukon gold potatoes, peeled and cut into 1-in. cubes	Cold water
1 tsp. salt	2 TB. dairy-free margarine
	¼ cup soy creamer, warmed
	Freshly ground pepper

Yield: 6 servings

Prep time: 10 minutes

Cook time: 15 minutes

Serving size: about ½ cup

1. Place potatoes in a large pot, add salt and enough cold water to cover, and bring to a boil over high heat.

2. Reduce heat to medium, and simmer potatoes for about 12 minutes or until fork-tender. Pour into a colander and allow to drain for 10 minutes.

3. Transfer potatoes to a large mixing bowl, and add margarine and warm soy creamer. Mash potatoes by hand to desired consistency, and season with freshly ground pepper. Serve immediately.

Dairy Don't _____

Restaurant-prepared mashed potatoes are almost always off-limits for dairy-free eaters because professional chefs and cooks routinely add butter and milk or cream.

Thanksgiving Candied Yams

Butter takes a holiday in this sweetly delectable favorite side dish flavored with brown sugar and maple syrup.

Yield: 6 to 8 servings	
Prep time: 10 minutes	
Cook time: 35 minutes	
Serving size: about ½ cup	

4 medium sweet potatoes, baked to fork-tender

Salt and pepper

⅓ cup dark corn syrup

¼ cup maple syrup

¼ cup firmly packed dark brown sugar

Marshmallows (optional)

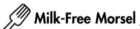 **Milk-Free Morsel**

Baking sweet potatoes instead of boiling them eliminates excess moisture when you want to use them for candied sweet potatoes and casseroles. Baking provides a wonderful caramelized flavor as well.

1. Preheat the oven to 375°F. Lightly coat a 9×13-inch baking dish with vegetable oil.

2. While potatoes are still warm, carefully remove skins using a paring knife. Cut into large cubes and place in a single layer in the prepared baking dish. Season with salt and pepper.

3. In a small saucepan, stir together corn syrup, maple syrup, and brown sugar. Cook over medium heat, stirring often, for 3 minutes or until sugar has dissolved.

4. Pour syrup mixture over sweet potatoes, and bake, basting occasionally, for 30 minutes or until potatoes are nicely glazed and bubbly. Top with marshmallows (if using) during the last 5 minutes.

5. Remove from the oven and allow to rest for 5 minutes before serving.

Whipped Sweet Potato Casserole

A great change from candied yams, this sweet casserole, fragrant with autumn spices and topped with a nutty cinnamon crunch, will have diners coming back for more.

4 medium sweet potatoes, baked to fork-tender

2 TB. dairy-free margarine, melted

2 large eggs, lightly beaten

2 TB. firmly packed light brown sugar

1 tsp. ground cinnamon

½ tsp. ground ginger

½ tsp. salt

¼ tsp. ground nutmeg

1 cup coarsely chopped pecans

1 TB. sugar

Yield: 6 to 8 servings
Prep time: 15 minutes
Cook time: 35 minutes
Serving size: about ½ cup

1. Preheat the oven to 350°F. Lightly coat a 9×13-inch glass casserole dish with margarine.

2. Remove skins from sweet potatoes using a paring knife and place pulp in a large mixing bowl. Add melted margarine, eggs, brown sugar, ½ teaspoon cinnamon, ginger, salt, and nutmeg.

3. Using an electric mixer on medium speed, beat sweet potato mixture for 2 minutes or until smooth. Transfer to the prepared casserole dish, and spread evenly.

4. In a small mixing bowl, stir together pecans, sugar, and remaining ½ teaspoon cinnamon. Sprinkle over top of casserole, and bake for 30 to 35 minutes or until puffed up and slightly golden around the edges. Serve immediately.

Free Fact

Myriad species and cultivars of cinnamon are grown around the world, but "true cinnamon" is considered Ceylon cinnamon, which is milder than its spicy relatives.

Buttery Baked Acorn Squash

Calcium-rich sesame seeds and a spoonful of brown sugar add flavor and interest to this terrific healthy side dish.

2 medium acorn squash, halved lengthwise, seeds removed	**4 tsp. dairy-free margarine**
	4 heaping tsp. brown sugar
	1½ tsp. sesame seeds

> *Yield: 4 servings*
>
> **Prep time:** 15 minutes
> **Cook time:** 50 minutes
> **Serving size:** ½ acorn squash

1. Preheat the oven to 375°F. Pour 1 cup of water in a 9×13-inch roasting pan.

2. Place the halved squash flesh side down in the roasting pan and bake for 30 minutes.

3. Using tongs, turn over the squash halves and place a teaspoon of margarine and brown sugar into each cavity. Return to the oven and bake for 10 minutes.

4. Brush the melted margarine and sugar over the flesh of the squash and sprinkle the sesame seeds over. Continue to bake for 10 minutes more or until the flesh is fork tender and the squash has begun to brown.

5. Remove from the oven and allow to rest 5 minutes before serving.

Free Fact

Acorn squash are a good source of beta-carotene, dietary fiber, and potassium. They can be stored for several months in a cool, dry location.

Green Bean–Mushroom Casserole

If you thought this old favorite was off-limits, think again. This creamy, rich version made from flavorful fresh ingredients will win any taste test.

1 lb. fresh green beans, trimmed and cooked to fork-tender, or 1 lb. frozen green beans, cooked according to pkg. directions

1 TB. vegetable oil

1 tsp. dairy-free margarine

8 oz. sliced white mushrooms

Salt and pepper

1 garlic clove, minced

1½ TB. all-purpose flour

¾ cup low-sodium chicken or vegetable broth

½ cup soy creamer

1 (3-oz.) can french-fried onions

> *Yield: 6 servings*
> **Prep time:** 15 minutes
> **Cook time:** 30 minutes
> **Serving size:** about ½ cup

1. Preheat the oven to 425°F. Lightly coat a 1-quart casserole with 1 teaspoon dairy-free margarine.

2. Pat dry cooked green beans with a paper towel and place in a large mixing bowl.

3. In a medium skillet over medium-high heat, heat vegetable oil with margarine. Add mushrooms, season with salt and pepper, and cook, stirring occasionally, for about 5 minutes or until lightly browned. Add garlic, and cook 1 more minute.

4. Sprinkle flour over mushrooms, and cook, stirring, for 1 minute. While continuing to stir, pour in chicken broth and soy creamer. Reduce heat to low, and simmer for about 5 minutes or until thickened.

5. Add mushroom mixture to green beans, and toss well to coat. Transfer to the prepared casserole, sprinkle french-fried onions over top, and bake for 15 minutes or until heated through and just beginning to bubble. Serve immediately.

Free Fact

Now a beloved side dish with many variations, the original green bean casserole recipe was created by Campbell's Soup in 1955 to help sell cans of their cream of mushroom soup.

Crumb-Topped Broccoli Bake

Dairy-free sour cream steps in for a hint of creaminess in this easy and scrumptious broccoli side featuring the flavor of Italian herbs.

Yield: 4 servings
Prep time: 10 minutes
Cook time: 12 minutes
Serving size: 1 cup

4 cups broccoli florets

Juice of ½ lemon

Salt and pepper

¼ cup dairy-free sour cream

⅓ cup plain breadcrumbs

2 tsp. dried Italian herb blend

Olive oil

1. Bring a large pot of salted water to a boil over high heat. Add broccoli, and cook for 5 to 8 minutes or until fork-tender. Drain and transfer to a 1-quart ovenproof casserole dish.

2. Preheat the broiler.

3. Drizzle lemon juice over broccoli, and season with salt and pepper. Spread sour cream on top.

4. In a small bowl, combine breadcrumbs and Italian herb blend. Sprinkle over sour cream, and drizzle olive oil over breadcrumbs.

5. Place under the broiler for about 2 minutes or until breadcrumbs have browned and sour cream has melted. Serve immediately.

Milk-Free Morsel

Broccoli, a member of the cruciferous family, is an excellent source of calcium. Add it to soups and casseroles, and serve it raw in salads and on vegetable dip platters.

Sautéed Spinach with Garlic

Nutritious spinach takes center stage in this Mediterranean-style preparation flavored with pungent garlic.

2 TB. extra-virgin olive oil

3 garlic cloves, roughly chopped

4 cups baby spinach, washed and dried

¼ cup low-sodium chicken or vegetable broth

Salt and pepper

Yield: 4 servings	
Prep time: 5 minutes	
Cook time: 5 minutes	
Serving size: ½ cup	

1. In a large, nonstick skillet over medium heat, heat olive oil. Add garlic, and cook for 1 minute or until fragrant but not browned.

2. Add spinach in handfuls, stirring after each addition. Pour in chicken broth, and continue to cook, stirring, for about 2 more minutes or until spinach has wilted and liquid has evaporated.

3. Season with salt and pepper, and serve immediately.

 Milk-Free Morsel

> Instead of serving vegetables boiled and buttered, start sautéing them in healthy olive oil and garlic for terrific flavor and dairy-free results.

Oven-Roasted Parma Cauliflower

A terrific departure from the usual cauliflower with cheese sauce, this oven-roasted version gets its flavor from caramelized browning and a hint of vegan Parmesan cheese.

Yield: 4 servings
Prep time: 12 minutes
Cook time: 25 minutes
Serving size: 1 cup

1 medium head cauliflower, leaves removed

2 TB. extra-virgin olive oil

Salt and pepper

1 TB. vegan Parmesan cheese

1. Preheat the oven to 375°F.

2. Remove tough core from cauliflower and break into large florets. Cut each floret into ¼-inch-thick slices, and arrange on a large rimmed baking sheet coated lightly with olive oil.

3. Drizzle extra-virgin olive oil over cauliflower, and season with salt and pepper. Roast, occasionally shaking the pan to brown evenly, for about 25 minutes or until tender and golden on the edges.

4. Remove from the oven and sprinkle with vegan Parmesan cheese. Allow to rest for 3 minutes before serving.

Free Fact

Cauliflower with cheese sauce is actually a British creation often served as a main dish and called simply "cauliflower cheese." Make your own dairy-free version using Cheezy Cream Sauce (recipe in Chapter 16).

Zesty Lemon-Asparagus Hollandaise

No need to do without this luxurious dish, rich with buttery flavor. Crisp asparagus and tangy lemon create the perfect foil for a heavenly blanket of flavor.

1 lb. medium-thickness asparagus spears, woody stems removed

Pinch salt

Water

1 tsp. lemon zest

Freshly ground pepper

1 batch Dairy-Free Hollandaise (recipe in Chapter 16), warm

Yield: 4 servings	
Prep time: 10 minutes	
Cook time: 5 minutes	
Serving size: 4 or 5 spears	

1. Wash asparagus spears and place in a microwave-safe dish. Add salt and 1 tablespoon water, cover, and microwave on high for 5 minutes or until crisp-tender.

2. Transfer spears to a warmed serving platter. Sprinkle with lemon zest and season with pepper.

3. Pour warm Dairy-Free Hollandaise over all, and serve immediately.

Free Fact

Microplane zesters are great for obtaining the essence of citrus zest without the bitter white pith.

Chapter 15

Rice, Beans, and Grains

In This Chapter

- ◆ Sensational, substantial sides
- ◆ Beans make the dish
- ◆ Delicious, dairy-free grain creations

Sometimes a fantastic side dish can really make the meal, particularly when it's full of substance and flavor. The side dishes in this chapter fit that description perfectly. Some unusual dairy-free ingredients provide yummy flavor, while a rich and creamy texture is the result of some surprising additions.

Creating dishes using healthful beans and grains is another way to keep the element of delightful surprise at the dinner table. No one will be able to resist reaching for a second helping of these nutritious, delicious sides, so start expanding your side dish repertoire by diving into the fabulous recipes that follow.

"Cheesy" Rice Pilaf with Peas

Nutritional yeast flakes provide a hint of cheese in this delectable side dish that's full of flavor.

Yield: 4 servings
Prep time: 12 minutes
Cook time: 25 minutes
Serving size: 1 cup

1 TB. dairy-free margarine

1 small onion, minced

Salt and pepper

1 cup long-grain white rice

1 cup low-sodium chicken or vegetable broth

1¼ cups water

2 TB. nutritional yeast flakes

⅔ cup frozen green peas, thawed

1. In a medium saucepan over medium heat, melt margarine. Add onion, salt, and pepper, and sauté for about 3 minutes or until onion is soft. Stir in rice to coat.

2. Pour in chicken broth and water, stir well to combine, and bring to a boil. Cover, reduce heat to low, and cook for 20 minutes.

3. Remove from heat and stir in nutritional yeast flakes and peas. Allow to sit, covered, for 5 minutes before fluffing with a fork and serving.

⊘ Dairy Don't _____

Restaurant rice pilafs as well as those made from other grains are usually heavy on the butter and sometimes cream and cheese as well. If offered as a side dish when dining out, ask for plain, steamed rice instead.

Southwest Red Beans and Rice

Piquant chili powder and cumin highlight this delicious rice side, while creamy red beans provide a good dose of protein.

2 cups water	1 cup tomato sauce
1 cup long-grain white rice	1 (16-oz.) can red kidney beans, drained and rinsed
¾ tsp. salt	
1 TB. chili powder	Dairy-free sour cream (optional)
1 tsp. ground cumin	1 TB. chopped fresh cilantro leaves (optional)
½ tsp. paprika	

Yield: 4 servings

Prep time: 10 minutes
Cook time: 25 minutes
Serving size: 1 cup

1. In a medium saucepan over high heat, bring water to a boil. Stir in rice, salt, chili powder, cumin, and paprika. Reduce heat to low, cover, and cook for 20 minutes.

2. Stir in tomato sauce and beans, increase heat to medium, and cook, stirring often, for about 5 minutes or until piping hot.

3. Transfer to a serving bowl, and top with dollop of sour cream (if using) and chopped cilantro (if using). Serve immediately.

Milk-Free Morsel

Use leftover plain cooked rice to create a quick and hearty rice and bean dish by heating it with tomato sauce and seasonings in a skillet and adding your choice of beans just to heat through.

Brown Rice Tabbouleh

Terrific hot or cold, this variation on a healthy side dish fragrant with fresh mint and finished with the tang of soy yogurt is great with grilled lamb or chicken.

Yield: 6 servings
Prep time: 15 minutes
Cook time: 45 minutes
Serving size: about ¾ cup

1 TB. dairy-free margarine

1 TB. olive oil

4 scallions, trimmed and sliced

½ green bell pepper, seeded, cored, and diced small

1 cup brown rice

2½ cups low-sodium chicken or vegetable broth

Juice of ½ lemon

¼ cup finely chopped fresh mint leaves

¼ cup finely chopped fresh parsley leaves

Salt and pepper

8 oz. plain soy yogurt

1. Melt together margarine and olive oil in a medium saucepan over medium heat. Add scallions and bell pepper and cook, stirring occasionally, for 3 minutes until slightly softened.

2. Add brown rice and stir well to coat the grains. Add broth, bring to a boil, reduce heat to low, cover, and cook for 40 to 45 minutes until the rice is tender, adding a bit of water if necessary.

3. Remove from heat and let stand covered for 5 minutes.

4. Add lemon, mint, and parsley and fluff with a fork to combine. Season with salt and pepper, and serve immediately or allow to cool and serve topped with dollops of yogurt.

 Milk-Free Morsel

Keep fresh herbs at peak freshness by wrapping a damp paper towel around the stems of the bunch and storing in the crisper drawer of your refrigerator.

Spicy Refried Black Beans

This favorite Mexican side full of important protein gets a kick from fresh jalapeño peppers and a finish from creamy melted nondairy cheese.

1 TB. vegetable oil	¼ cup water
½ small onion, minced	¼ tsp. ground cumin
1 jalapeño pepper, seeds removed, and minced	Salt and pepper
1 (16-oz.) can black beans, drained and rinsed	½ cup shredded dairy-free cheddar cheese

Yield: 4 servings
Prep time: 10 minutes
Cook time: 15 minutes
Serving size: ½ cup

1. Preheat the oven to 400°F.

2. In a medium nonstick skillet over medium heat, heat vegetable oil. Add onion and jalapeño, and cook, stirring often, for 3 or 4 minutes or until softened.

3. Add black beans, water, and cumin. Continue cooking, stirring occasionally, for 3 more minutes.

4. Remove from heat, and using a potato masher or the back of a spoon, coarsely mash bean mixture to paste. Season with salt and pepper, and spread out in an 8-inch shallow pie plate.

5. Top with cheese, and bake for about 8 minutes or until cheese has melted and beans are piping hot. Serve immediately.

Free Fact

Black beans, also called black turtle beans, are the most popular bean used in Latin American cuisine. It is not the same black bean used in Asian black bean paste, which actually utilizes a type of fermented black soybean.

Curried Dahl with Lentils

An Indian staple, dahl gets its creamy consistency from lentils in this spicy version that's a protein powerhouse of exotic flavor.

Yield: *4 servings*
Prep time: 10 minutes
Cook time: 25 minutes
Serving size: about 1 cup

1 TB. vegetable oil

2 garlic cloves, minced

1 TB. finely chopped peeled fresh ginger

2 tsp. curry powder

¼ tsp. ground coriander

¼ tsp. ground cumin

Dash cayenne

1 cup red lentils, rinsed

2 cups water

1 cup low-sodium chicken or vegetable broth

1 TB. tomato paste

Salt

Soy yogurt

1. In a medium saucepan over medium heat, heat vegetable oil. Add garlic and ginger, and cook, stirring often, for 1 minute without browning.

2. Stir in curry powder, coriander, cumin, and cayenne, and cook 30 more seconds.

3. Add lentils, water, and chicken broth, and stir to combine. Bring to a boil, reduce heat to low, and cook, stirring occasionally, for 13 to 15 minutes or until lentils are softened.

4. Stir in tomato paste, and season with salt. Continue to cook 5 more minutes or until creamy and thick.

5. Serve by the spoonful with dollop of soy yogurt on top.

🚫 **Dairy Don't**

Indian restaurants often finish dahls and stews with a dollop of yogurt for smoothness and richness. Be sure to ask when dining out.

Boy Oh Boy Arborio Risotto

Who doesn't love the creamy richness of a real risotto? Butternut squash and a touch of soy make this dairy-free version the most delicious and creamiest yet.

2 TB. dairy-free margarine	¼ tsp. ground nutmeg
1 TB. olive oil	1 cup *Arborio rice*
1 small onion, minced	¼ cup apple juice
1 cup butternut squash, peeled, seeded, and cut into small dice	1 qt. low-sodium chicken or vegetable broth, kept hot on the back burner
Salt and pepper	¼ cup soy creamer

Yield: 4 servings
Prep time: 15 minutes
Cook time: 30 minutes
Serving size: about ¾ cup

1. In a large saucepan over medium heat, melt together margarine and oil. Add onion and butternut squash, season with salt and pepper, and cook, stirring often, for about 5 minutes until onion has softened.

2. Add nutmeg and rice, and cook over medium-high heat, stirring constantly, for 1 minute. Stir in apple juice and cook a further minute.

3. Using a ½ cup ladle, begin adding hot broth to rice, stirring constantly each time, until liquid has been absorbed. Be sure to keep rice at a low simmer while stirring.

4. When all broth has been used, add soy creamer and continue stirring and cooking over low heat until rice is tender and creamy but still firm to the bite.

5. Remove from the heat and serve immediately.

Lactose Lingo

Arborio rice is an Italian short grain rice named after the town where it is grown. Its round, chewy, and starchy consistency are ideal for risotto.

Creamy Barley Risotto

Nutritious and nutty, barley creates its own rich consistency in this delicious dairy-free version of a restaurant favorite.

🌾 🫛

Yield: 4 servings
Prep time: 10 minutes
Cook time: 50 minutes
Serving size: 1 cup

2 tsp. dairy-free margarine

1 medium onion, finely chopped

Salt and pepper

1 cup pearl barley

2 tsp. chopped fresh thyme leaves

½ cup white wine or white grape juice

4 cups chicken or vegetable broth

¼ cup soy creamer

1 TB. chopped fresh parsley leaves

1. In a large nonstick skillet over medium heat, melt margarine. Add onion, season with salt and pepper, and cook for 4 minutes or until softened.

2. Add barley and thyme, and stir to combine. Pour in wine or grape juice, and cook for 2 or 3 minutes or until liquid is absorbed.

3. Stir in 2 cups chicken broth, and bring mixture to a boil. Reduce heat to low, and simmer for about 5 minutes or until most of liquid is absorbed.

4. Continue to add broth to barley mixture, ½ cup at a time, stirring often and waiting to add more broth until absorbed. Cook a total of 40 minutes or until barley is tender and mixture is creamy.

5. Stir in soy creamer, remove from heat, and serve by the spoonful topped with chopped fresh parsley.

Free Fact _____

Barley is a member of the grass family, and although it's a common ingredient in malting and many healthful products such as barley water, it's primarily grown for animal feed.

Quinoa with Cashews

The naturally nutty flavor of this unusual grain teams up with delicious cashews and a hint of cilantro for a tasty side dish.

1 cup *quinoa*	**1 bay leaf**
2 TB. olive oil	**½ tsp. ground coriander**
1 medium celery stalk, trimmed and diced small	**½ tsp. ground cumin**
½ red bell pepper, seeded, cored, and diced small	**¼ tsp. ground ginger**
	¼ tsp. turmeric
Salt and pepper	**1¾ cup water**
½ cup raw cashews	**2 TB. finely chopped fresh parsley leaves**

Yield: 6 servings

Prep time: 15 minutes
Cook time: 25 minutes
Serving size: about ⅔ cup

1. Soak quinoa in cold water for 5 minutes. Rinse and set aside to drain.

2. In a medium saucepan heat olive oil over medium heat, add celery and red bell pepper, season with salt and pepper, and cook, stirring occasionally, for 5 minutes, until softened.

3. Stir in cashews, bay leaf, coriander, cumin, ginger, and turmeric and continue cooking for 2 minutes.

4. Add quinoa and cook, stirring frequently, for 2 minutes until dry. Pour in water and bring to a boil.

5. Reduce the heat to low, cover, and cook for about 15 minutes, until the water is absorbed and the grains are tender.

6. Remove from the heat, add parsley and fluff with a fork. Serve immediately.

Lactose Lingo

Quinoa is a gluten-free grain originating in Peru and is an excellent source of protein and dietary fiber. It should always be soaked and rinsed to remove the protective bitter coating called saponins.

Corny Cornbread Stuffing

The perfect savory stuffing for poultry, this side dish made from dairy-free corn muffins is deliciously fragrant with fresh sage and marjoram.

O ⚕ ⌒

Yield: 8 servings	
Prep time: 15 minutes	
Cook time: 45 minutes	
Serving size: about 1 cup	

1 batch Corn Muffins (recipe in Chapter 5), cut into cubes

2 TB. dairy-free margarine

1 large onion, diced

1 large celery stalk, diced

Salt and pepper

1 cup canned corn kernels, drained

1 medium red delicious apple, cored and diced

1 TB. chopped fresh sage leaves

1 tsp. dried sage leaves

1 tsp. dried marjoram

1 large egg, slightly beaten

1 cup low-sodium chicken or vegetable broth

1. Preheat the oven to 350°F. Lightly coat a 9×13-inch baking pan with dairy-free margarine.

2. Place cubed Corn Muffins on a baking sheet, and toast in the oven for 10 minutes. Transfer to a large mixing bowl, and set aside.

3. In a large nonstick skillet over medium-high heat, melt margarine. Add onion and celery, and season with salt and pepper. Cook, stirring occasionally, for about 3 minutes or until softened.

4. Stir in corn, apple, fresh sage, dried sage, and marjoram, and continue to cook, stirring often, for 2 minutes. Remove from heat, and add to the mixing bowl with Corn Muffin cubes. Toss gently to combine.

5. Stir in egg and chicken broth, transfer to the prepared pan, and bake, covered with foil, for 35 minutes or until firm and heated through.

Free Fact

"Shelled" corn was so named because early settlers noticed that Native Americans removed the corn from cobs by using a clamshell.

Nutty Wild Rice Stuffing

A wonderful alternative to bread stuffing, nutty wild rice pairs well with sweet dried cranberries and pecans for a fabulous side full of texture and flavor.

Yield: 6 servings
Prep time: 10 minutes
Cook time: 70 minutes
Serving size: about ⅔ cup

1 cup wild rice, rinsed	Salt and pepper
2 cups water	½ cup dried cranberries
1 cup low-sodium chicken or vegetable broth	½ cup chopped pecans
1 TB. olive oil	¼ cup cranberry juice
1 medium onion, diced	¼ cup chopped fresh parsley leaves
1 garlic clove, minced	1 large egg, slightly beaten

1. In a medium saucepan over high heat, combine wild rice, water, and chicken broth, and bring to a boil. Reduce heat to low and simmer, covered, for about 40 minutes or until wild rice is tender. Drain and transfer to a large mixing bowl.

2. Preheat the oven to 325°F. Lightly coat a 9×13-inch baking pan with dairy-free margarine.

3. In a medium nonstick skillet over medium heat, heat olive oil. Add onion and cook, stirring frequently, for about 3 minutes or until onion is softened. Stir in garlic, salt, pepper, cranberries, and pecans, and cook 1 more minute.

4. Add cranberry juice to the skillet, and cook for about 30 seconds or until absorbed. Transfer mixture to the bowl with wild rice, add parsley and egg, and stir well to combine.

5. Transfer stuffing to the prepared baking pan, and bake, covered with foil, for about 25 minutes or until firm and heated through.

> ### Free Fact
> Unrelated to the rice family, wild rice is actually a type of grass grown in the shallow water of lakes. Minnesota is the largest producer of wild rice in the United States.

Chapter 16

Dairy-Free Sauces and Gravies

In This Chapter

- ◆ Gettin' saucy, without the dairy
- ◆ Delicious dairy-free condiments
- ◆ Consistently creamy gravies

Many enjoy the decadence of a rich and creamy sauce or gravy, but too often the addition of dairy makes these delicious extras taboo. If it's been a long while since you've relished a creamy white sauce or a rich pan gravy, your wait is over. Obtaining creamy results is not limited to the inclusion of cream. Simple roux made with dairy-free margarine or oil and flour can create the richest sauces and gravies around. Deep, rich flavor is doable when you know the right ingredients to include, from fresh herbs to earthy mushrooms. Fantastically faux, with unbelievable flavor, the recipes in this chapter put sauce back on the menu.

Many condiments in the supermarket, from tartar sauce to tzatziki, may actually contain hidden dairy, so why not whip up your own healthy versions using the recipes in this chapter? You'll be amazed how easy it is and how great you feel when you eliminate the unwanted dairy.

Beautiful Béchamel

The classic creamy white sauce gets a dairy-free makeover in this version that features unsweetened soy milk and a hint of cayenne and nutmeg.

Yield: 2 cups
Prep time: 5 minutes
Cook time: 8 minutes
Serving size: about ¼ to ½ cup

3 TB. dairy-free margarine	**Dash cayenne**
3 TB. all-purpose flour	**Dash nutmeg**
2 cups unsweetened soy milk	**¼ cup soy creamer**
Salt	

1. In a medium saucepan over medium heat, melt margarine. Add flour, and whisk to combine. Cook for 1 or 2 minutes, whisking constantly, until large bubbles form. Do not brown.

2. Slowly add soy milk, continuing to whisk as sauce thickens for 3 or 4 minutes. Add salt, cayenne, and nutmeg, and cook for 1 more minute. Sauce should be a consistency to coat the back of a spoon.

3. Remove from heat and whisk in soy creamer. Taste for additional seasoning, and use immediately or cover and cool before storing in the refrigerator for up to 2 days.

 Milk-Free Morsel

When reheating creamy sauces, be sure to use a low flame and avoid boiling. Whisking rather than stirring ensures a smooth, creamy result.

"Cheezy" Cream Sauce

Turn your creamy béchamel into this tangy "cheezy" cream sauce perfect for adding zip to plain veggies or pasta.

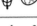

2 cups Beautiful Béchamel (recipe earlier in this chapter)

6 TB. nutritional yeast flakes

½ cup shredded dairy-free cheddar cheese

½ tsp. mustard

Dash ground turmeric

Yield: about 2 cups
Prep time: 5 minutes
Cook time: 6 minutes
Serving size: about ¼ to ½ cup

1. In a medium saucepan over low heat, warm Beautiful Béchamel.

2. Add nutritional yeast flakes, and whisk for about 2 minutes or until well combined and bubbly.

3. Switch to a wooden spoon for stirring, and add cheddar cheese, mustard, and turmeric.

4. Stir constantly for about 2 more minutes or until cheese has melted. Serve immediately, or cover and cool before storing in the refrigerator for up to 2 days.

Milk-Free Morsel

You might find lactose-free or lactose-reduced cheeses in your supermarket's dairy department. If milk allergies aren't a concern, give these products a try.

Dairy-Free Hollandaise

Unbelievably delicious and rich, with an amazing buttery flavor, this version fills in perfectly for the original on vegetables or poached eggs.

Yield: about 2 cups
Prep time: 10 minutes
Cook time: 5 minutes
Serving size: about ¼ to ½ cup

4 large egg yolks	**Salt and pepper**
1 TB. lemon juice	**½ cup (1 stick) dairy-free margarine, melted and kept warm**
½ tsp. dry mustard	

1. In a medium mixing bowl, combine egg yolks, lemon juice, mustard, salt, and pepper. With an electric mixer on high speed, beat for about 3 minutes or until yolk mixture becomes light yellow and ribbony. Transfer to the top of a double boiler.

2. Whisk yolk mixture as it heats, and slowly add warm, melted margarine in a stream. Whisk constantly until thick and piping hot. Serve immediately.

⊘ Dairy Don't _____

If you're tempted by convenience and want to try using prepared sauce packets with dairy-free margarine instead of butter, be aware that milk derivatives may be present in the powder. Read labels carefully.

Garlic and Herb Sauce

Here's a creamy and versatile sauce that will liven up vegetables, chicken, or pasta with the bold flavor of garlic and the intoxicating fragrance of fresh herbs.

1 (8-oz.) package silken tofu, drained	2 tsp. chopped fresh parsley leaves
1½ cups soy milk	2 tsp. chopped fresh dill
2 TB. dairy-free margarine	Salt and pepper
3 large garlic cloves, minced	1 TB. cornstarch
1 TB. nutritional yeast flakes	3 TB. water
2 tsp. chopped fresh basil leaves	

Yield: 4 to 6 servings
Prep time: 10 minutes
Cook time: 5 minutes
Serving size: about ½ cup

1. In a food processor fitted with a steel blade, purée the tofu 1 minute until smooth.

2. Add soy milk, margarine, garlic, nutritional yeast, basil, parsley, and dill. Process 1 minute until smooth and well combined.

3. Pour the mixture into a medium saucepan, season with salt and pepper, and cook, stirring, over medium heat until bubbly.

4. In a small bowl stir together cornstarch and water and add to the sauce while stirring. Continue to cook at a low simmer, stirring constantly, for 2 minutes until the sauce is thickened.

5. Remove from the heat and serve immediately.

 Milk-Free Morsel

Whenever you are using cornstarch as a thickener it is always necessary to allow the mixture to boil for at least one minute in order for the cornstarch to reach its full thickening power.

Quick Tartar Sauce

This homemade tartar sauce removes any worries of added milk products bottled versions might contain, while featuring fresh aromatic herbs and the wonderfully piquant flavor of pickles and capers.

Yield: about 1 cup
Prep time: 30 minutes
Serving size: 1 tablespoon

1 cup mayonnaise

1 TB. lemon juice

1 TB. capers, drained and chopped

2 TB. chopped sweet pickles

2 tsp. finely chopped fresh parsley leaves

1 tsp. finely chopped fresh tarragon leaves

Dash hot pepper sauce

1. In a small bowl, stir together mayonnaise, lemon juice, capers, sweet pickles, parsley, tarragon, and hot pepper sauce.

2. Transfer to an airtight container, and refrigerate for 15 minutes before using. Keep refrigerated for up to 3 days.

Free Fact

Tartar sauce, a French condiment originally created to accompany steak tartar, a raw chopped beef dish, is named after the early Russian clan of Tatars, who were known for their rather barbaric culinary sense of preferring raw over cooked meat.

Soy Yogurt Tzatziki

This delicious Greek-style condiment with the alluring flavors of fresh mint and garlic is perfect as an accompaniment to fish or a topping for falafel or grilled veggies.

2 cups plain soy yogurt

1 small cucumber, peeled, seeds removed, and diced

2 tsp. lime juice

Salt and pepper

2 garlic cloves, minced

2 TB. chopped fresh mint leaves

Yield: About 2 cups
Prep time: 1 hour, 50 minutes
Serving size: 2 table-spoons

1. Line a strainer with cheesecloth and place over a bowl. Add yogurt and allow to drain in the refrigerator for 1 hour.

2. In a medium bowl, combine drained yogurt, cucumber, lime juice, salt, pepper, garlic, and mint. Stir well and refrigerate for 30 minutes before using. Transfer to an airtight container and keep refrigerated for up to 3 days.

 Milk-Free Morsel

Tzatziki is also a great choice for a vegetable dip, particularly at kids' parties, where milk allergies may be common.

Quick and Creamy Gravy

Delicious when made from scratch or from your own pan drippings, this easy gravy full of flavor and richness is perfect for poultry or biscuits.

Yield: about 2 cups
Prep time: 10 minutes
Cook time: 10 minutes
Serving size: 3 table-spoons

¼ cup (½ stick) dairy-free margarine or pan drippings

1 small onion, finely chopped

Salt and pepper

¼ cup all-purpose flour

1 cup low-sodium chicken broth

¾ cup unsweetened soy milk

Pinch dried thyme

2 TB. soy creamer

1. In a medium nonstick skillet over medium-high heat, melt margarine. Add onion, season with salt and pepper, and cook, stirring frequently, for about 2 minutes or until lightly browned.

2. Sprinkle flour over onion and cook, stirring to combine, for 1 more minute. Pour in chicken broth and soy milk, increase heat to high, and whisk constantly for about 5 minutes or until thickened.

3. Stir in thyme and soy creamer, taste for additional seasoning, and serve immediately.

⊘ Dairy Don't _____

Jarred or canned gravies can contain milk protein in many forms. Take care when eating out as well, because cooks often use powdered thickeners even in preparations made from scratch.

Delectable Mushroom Gravy

Thick and rich, with the earthy flavor of mushrooms and hearty beef broth, this gravy pairs well with everything from meatloaf to roast beef.

8 oz. white or baby bella mushrooms

¼ cup (½ stick) dairy-free margarine or pan drippings

Salt and pepper

1 garlic clove, minced

¼ cup all-purpose flour

1½ cups low-sodium beef broth

½ tsp. dried parsley

2 TB. soy creamer

Yield: about 2 cups
Prep time: 15 minutes
Cook time: 12 minutes
Serving size: 3 table-spoons

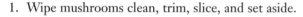

1. Wipe mushrooms clean, trim, slice, and set aside.

2. In a medium nonstick skillet over medium-high heat, melt margarine. Add mushrooms, season with salt and pepper, and cook, stirring occasionally, for 4 to 6 minutes or until lightly browned. Stir in garlic, and cook for 1 more minute.

3. Add flour and cook, stirring constantly, for 1 more minute. Pour in beef broth, increase heat to high, and whisk constantly for about 5 minutes or until thickened.

4. Stir in parsley and soy creamer, taste for additional seasoning, and serve immediately.

Milk-Free Morsel

Freeze extra homemade gravy to take along to family holiday gatherings, to be sure you're not left out when the host's potentially dairy-containing gravy is ladled up.

Part 5

Amazing Desserts

For many people, Part 5 might be the ultimate test of whether dairy-free cooking is really up to snuff. When it comes to dessert, making substitutions for beloved dairy ingredients like butter and cream might even prompt the least skeptical among us to question the outcome. Well, get ready to be shocked and awed by some amazing desserts.

If crisp, buttery cookies are your passion, don't worry. If fudgy, rich brownies get you excited, be prepared. Never mind the cakes, pies, and puddings that await. And perhaps the most surprising reaction of all will be when you take your first spoonful of ultrasmooth, purely decadent dairy-free ice cream. Even the toughest customers will have to agree that life without dairy is no longer a disagreeable prospect.

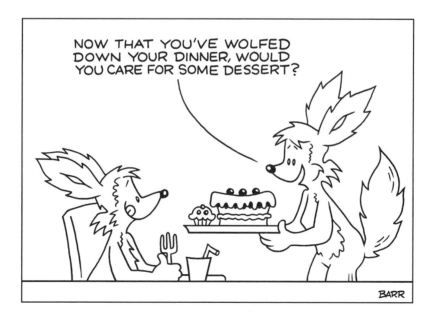

Chapter 17

Cookies, Brownies, and Cakes

In This Chapter

♦ A cookie jar of delectability

♦ Easy stand-ins for dairy-free baking

♦ Unusual ingredients yield delicious results

Soon after you dive into this chapter, you'll realize that delicious dairy-free desserts are just a baking sheet away. Cookies you thought could never be as good as their dairy-filled counterparts will disappear before you know it. Every cookie in this chapter is deliciously dairy free, and it will be hard to eat just one when they emerge from the oven.

Finding substitutes for dessert baking isn't difficult. Margarines work as well as butter in recipes from cookies, to brownies, to cakes, while cow's milk alternatives stand in extremely well and even add a bit of flavor of their own when included in the ingredient list. So rest assured you already have the substitutes you need to perfect your dairy-free baking techniques.

Occasionally, however, some rather unusual ingredients provide the answer to your dairy-free question. Delicious cookies and cake made with olive oil rather than butter will surprise and delight you. Cake flour and semolina contribute just the right texture for just the right cake, while dairy-free chocolate in many different forms proves that indulgence, not depravation, is on the menu.

Chewy Chocolate-Chip Cookies

No need to give up these irresistible creations when you follow this dairy-free recipe, packed with dark chocolate flavor and a deliciously chewy inside.

Yield: about 4 dozen

Prep time: 25 minutes

Cook time: 8 to 11 minutes

Serving size: 2 or 3 cookies

1 cup (2 sticks) dairy-free margarine, softened

¾ cup granulated sugar

¾ cup light or dark brown sugar, firmly packed

2 large eggs

1 tsp. vanilla extract

2¼ cups all-purpose flour

1 tsp. baking soda

1 tsp. salt

12 oz. dairy-free chocolate chips or chopped dark chocolate (about 1½ cups)

1. Preheat the oven to 375°F. Line a cookie sheet with parchment paper.

2. In a medium bowl, and using an electric mixer on high speed, beat margarine, granulated sugar, and brown sugar until creamy. Beat in eggs and vanilla extract until well combined.

3. Reduce mixer speed to medium and add flour, a little at a time. Add baking soda and salt, and beat for 1 more minute. Stir in chocolate until well combined.

4. Drop by tablespoonfuls onto the prepared cookie sheets about 2 inches apart.

5. Bake for 8 to 11 minutes or until edges are just golden and centers are still soft. Cool for 5 minutes on the cookie sheets, transfer cookies to wire racks to cool completely, and repeat with remaining dough. Keep stored in an airtight container for up to 5 days.

Dairy Don't

Selecting chocolate that has greater than 71 percent cocoa content usually guarantees no dairy ingredients are present. However, be sure to read labels carefully because some dark chocolate chips with lower percentages may actually be dairy free, while some bittersweet versions may not.

Cashew Butter Cookies

This variation on the traditional peanut butter cookie will surprise you with its intense cashew flavor and sweetly soft texture.

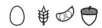

1 cup (2 sticks) dairy-free margarine, softened

1 cup cashew butter

1¼ cups light brown sugar, firmly packed

2 large eggs

1 tsp. vanilla extract

½ tsp. baking soda

¼ tsp. baking powder

½ tsp. salt

3 cups all-purpose flour

48 cashew halves

Yield: 4 dozen
Prep time: 20 minutes
Cook time: 11 to 13 minutes
Serving size: 2 or 3 cookies

1. Preheat the oven to 350°F. Line 2 cookie sheets with parchment paper.

2. In a large mixing bowl, and using an electric mixer on medium speed, beat margarine and cashew butter until fluffy. Beat in eggs and vanilla extract until smooth.

3. In another large bowl, whisk together baking soda, baking powder, salt, and flour. Add flour mixture to wet mixture in 3 batches, stirring well after each addition.

4. Roll heaping tablespoons of dough into balls and place 1 inch apart on the cookie sheets. Flatten slightly with the tines of a fork, and press 1 cashew half in the middle of each.

5. Bake for 11 to 13 minutes or until cookies begin to brown. Transfer cookies to a wire rack to cool, and repeat with remaining dough. Store cookies in an airtight container for up to 1 week.

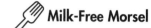

Milk-Free Morsel

Cashew butter, along with other nut butters, is increasingly available at supermarkets. Remember, though, for those with allergies, that store-ground nut butters could be cross-contacted with other allergens (e.g., peanuts) ground with the same equipment.

Open Sesame Meltaways

Healthful olive oil replaces butter in these soft, moderately sweet Mediterranean favorites with a hint of lemon and the crunch of sesame seeds.

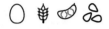

Yield: 5 dozen
Prep time: 15 minutes
Cook time: 15 to 18 minutes
Serving size: 4 or 5 cookies

½ cup light olive oil

½ cup (1 stick) dairy-free margarine, softened

¾ cup sugar

1 large egg

2 tsp. lemon juice

2½ cups all-purpose flour

¼ tsp. baking powder

¼ tsp. salt

½ cup soy milk

1 cup sesame seeds

1. Preheat the oven to 350°F. Line 2 cookie sheets with parchment paper.

2. In a large mixing bowl, and using an electric mixer on medium speed, beat olive oil, margarine, and sugar until smooth. Beat in egg and lemon juice until well combined.

3. In another bowl, whisk together flour, baking powder, and salt. Stir flour mixture into wet mixture in 2 batches. Dough will be smooth and soft.

4. Place soy milk in a small bowl and sesame seeds on a sheet of parchment paper. Scoop 1 tablespoon dough at a time and shape into a log. Dip in soy milk, roll in sesame seeds, and place on the cookie sheet 1 inch apart.

5. Bake for 15 to 18 minutes or until edges and bottoms are lightly toasted. Transfer cookies to a wire rack to cool, and repeat with remaining dough. Cookies will keep in an airtight container for up to 1 week.

Free Fact

The famous saying "Open, sesame!" from *Arabian Nights* refers to the bursting quality of a ripe sesame pod.

Grandma's Molasses Cookies

Chewy and moist, these terrific and flavorful cookies, loaded with tangy ginger and sharp molasses, are just like those found in Grandma's cookie jar.

¾ **cup vegetable oil**

1 cup sugar plus more for dipping

1 large egg

¼ **cup molasses**

2½ cups all-purpose flour

2 tsp. baking soda

1 tsp. ground cinnamon

1 tsp. ground ginger

½ **tsp. salt**

Yield: 3 dozen
Prep time: 15 minutes
Cook time: 7 to 9 minutes
Serving size: 2 cookies

1. Preheat the oven to 350°F. Line 2 cookie sheets with parchment paper.

2. In a large mixing bowl, and using an electric mixer on medium speed, beat vegetable oil, sugar, egg, and molasses until well combined.

3. In another bowl, whisk together flour, baking soda, cinnamon, ginger, and salt. Add dry ingredients in 2 batches to wet ingredients, stirring well each time to combine.

4. Scoop 1 tablespoon dough at a time and roll into balls. Dip in sugar, and place on the cookie sheet 2 inches apart.

5. Bake for 7 to 9 minutes or until cookies are lightly golden on the bottom and set. Transfer to a wire rack to cool, and repeat with remaining dough. Cookies will keep in an airtight container for up to 5 days.

Milk-Free Morsel

Freeze rolled balls of uncooked cookie dough for future small-batch cookie-baking. Allow to thaw in the refrigerator overnight before baking.

Iced Oatmeal Dunkers

Crisp and sweet with a thin coating of white icing, these terrific oatmeal cookies are great for dunking in vanilla soy or oat milk.

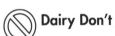

Yield: 4 dozen	

Prep time: 15 minutes
Cook time: 12 minutes
Serving size: 2 or 3 cookies

½ cup (1 stick) dairy-free margarine, softened

½ cup granulated sugar

½ cup dark brown sugar, firmly packed

1 large egg

½ tsp. vanilla extract

1 cup all-purpose flour

½ tsp. baking powder

½ tsp. baking soda

½ tsp. salt

½ tsp. ground cinnamon

¾ cup old-fashioned rolled oats

⅔ cup dark seedless raisins

2 cups confectioners' sugar

3 TB. vanilla soy milk

1. Preheat the oven to 350°F. Line 2 cookie sheets with parchment paper.

2. In a large bowl, and using an electric mixer on medium speed, beat margarine, granulated sugar, and brown sugar until fluffy. Add egg and vanilla extract, and beat until well combined.

3. In another bowl, whisk together flour, baking powder, baking soda, salt, and cinnamon. Add dry ingredients to wet ingredients in 2 batches, stirring well after each addition.

4. Stir in oats and raisins to combine.

5. Scoop 1 tablespoon dough at a time, and shape into ovals. Place on the cookie sheet, and flatten slightly with a metal spatula.

6. Bake for about 12 minutes or until cookies are lightly browned on edges. Transfer to a wire rack to cool completely, and repeat with remaining dough.

7. Make icing by whisking together confectioners' sugar and vanilla soy milk. Lightly spread over each cooled cookie, and return them to the wire rack until icing is set. Store in an airtight container for up to 1 week.

> **⊘ Dairy Don't** _____
>
> Glazes made from confectioners' sugar and cow's milk are common in supermarket bakeries, so read labels carefully on donuts, cinnamon buns, hot cross buns, cakes, and cookies.

Devil's Food Cake with Marshmallow Frosting

A classic combination gets a dairy-free makeover in this super-delicious chocolate cake topped with a light and fluffy, easy-to-make frosting.

⅔ cup dairy-free margarine, softened	1 tsp. salt
2 cups sugar	½ tsp. baking powder
3 large eggs	¾ cup cocoa powder
1½ tsp. vanilla extract	1⅓ cups cold water
2 cups all-purpose flour	2 TB. *meringue powder*
1¼ tsp. baking soda	¼ cup cold water
	½ cup light corn syrup

Yield: 1 (9-inch) layer cake, or 12 servings

Prep time: 20 minutes

Cook time: 30 to 35 minutes

Serving size: 1 slice

1. Preheat the oven to 350°F. Cut 2 circles of parchment paper to fit the bottom of 2 (9-inch) layer cake pans. Lightly coat the pans with dairy-free margarine and flour, knock out any excess flour, and place the parchment paper circles on the bottom.

2. In a medium bowl, and using an electric mixer on medium speed, beat margarine and 1⅔ cups sugar until light and fluffy. Beat in eggs 1 at a time, and add ½ teaspoon vanilla extract.

3. In another bowl, whisk together flour, baking soda, salt, and baking powder.

4. In another bowl, whisk together cocoa powder and cold water.

5. Alternate adding flour mixture and cocoa mixture to egg mixture in 2 batches, beating well after each addition. Pour into the prepared pans, and bake in the middle of the oven for 30 to 35 minutes or until a toothpick inserted in the center comes out clean.

6. Transfer to a wire rack to cool for 15 minutes. Remove cake from the pans, peel off the parchment paper, and allow cakes to cool completely on the rack.

7. In a medium bowl, and with an electric mixer on high speed, beat meringue powder and water for about 1 minute or until soft peaks form.

Lactose Lingo

Meringue powder is a popular professional baking ingredient made primarily of dehydrated egg whites. It is convenient and safe to use, particularly in recipes where raw egg whites might be called for.

8. Gradually beat in remaining ⅓ cup sugar for about 2 minutes or until stiff peaks form. Beat in remaining 1 teaspoon vanilla extract. Slowly pour corn syrup into meringue mixture while beating on high speed. Beat for about 3 more minutes or until frosting is thick and spreadable.

9. Place 1 cake layer top side down on a cake plate. Frost top with ⅓ of frosting, and top with other layer. Use remaining frosting to cover sides and top. Use the back of a teaspoon to make fluffy, marshmallowy peaks. Store frosted cake in a covered cake stand or carrier at room temperature for up to 4 days.

Moist Yellow Cake with "Butter" Cream Frosting

Sure to become the standard celebration cake in your house, this delicious dairy-free layer cake is topped with a rich and creamy buttery-flavored frosting.

²⁄₃ **cup plus ½ cup dairy-free margarine, softened**

1½ cups sugar

3 large eggs

3 tsp. vanilla extract

2½ cups *cake flour,* or 2¼ cups all-purpose flour

2½ tsp. baking powder

1 tsp. salt

½ cup unsweetened soy milk

½ cup soy creamer

4 cups confectioners' sugar

3 or 4 TB. vanilla soy milk

Yield: 1 (9-inch) layer cake, or 12 servings
Prep time: 20 minutes
Cook time: 25 to 30 minutes
Serving size: 1 slice

1. Preheat the oven to 350°F. Cut 2 circles of parchment paper to fit the bottom of 2 (9-inch) layer cake pans. Lightly coat the pans with dairy-free margarine and flour, knock out any excess flour, and place the parchment paper circles on the bottom.

2. In a medium bowl, and using an electric mixer on medium speed, beat ²⁄₃ cup margarine and sugar until light and fluffy. Beat in eggs one at a time, followed by 2 teaspoons vanilla extract.

3. In another bowl, whisk together flour, baking powder, and salt. Add flour mixture to wet mixture in 2 batches, beating well on medium speed after each addition. Beat in plain soy milk, followed by soy creamer.

4. Divide batter between the 2 prepared pans, and bake in the middle of the oven for 25 to 30 minutes or until tops are lightly golden and a toothpick inserted in the center comes out clean.

5. Let cool on a wire rack for 10 minutes, remove cakes from the pan, peel off the parchment, and let cakes cool completely on the wire racks.

> **Lactose Lingo**
>
> **Cake flour** is a soft, heavily milled wheat flour that's lower in protein than all-purpose flour and is preferred in cake baking when a tender crumb and light consistency are desired.

6. In a medium bowl, and using an electric mixer on high speed, beat remaining ½ cup margarine, confectioners' sugar, vanilla soy milk, and remaining 1 teaspoon vanilla extract. Add more soy milk as necessary to thin frosting, or more confectioners' sugar to make it spreadable.

7. When cakes are cool, place one layer top side down on a cake plate and frost with ⅓ of frosting. Place other layer, top side up, on top, and frost sides and top with remaining frosting. Cake will keep refrigerated for up to 5 days.

Coconut-Chocolate-Chip Blondies

Dotted with dark chocolate and oozing with flavor, these terrific cousins of brownies, sweetened with coconut and brown sugar, will delight every sweet tooth around.

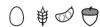

6 TB. dairy-free margarine, melted	2 tsp. baking powder
1¾ cups light brown sugar, firmly packed	½ tsp. salt
	¾ cup sweetened flaked coconut
2 large eggs	1 cup dairy-free chocolate chips or chopped dark chocolate
1 tsp. vanilla extract	
1 cup all-purpose flour	

Yield: 8 servings

Prep time: 15 minutes

Cook time: 25 to 30 minutes

Serving size: 2 blondies

1. Preheat the oven to 350°F. Lightly coat an 8×8-inch-square baking pan with margarine.

2. In a medium bowl, and using an electric mixer on medium speed, beat melted margarine and brown sugar. Add eggs and vanilla extract, and beat until well combined.

3. In another bowl, whisk together flour, baking powder, and salt. Add flour mixture to wet ingredients in 2 batches, stirring well to combine after each addition.

4. Stir in coconut and chocolate chips. Spread into the prepared baking pan, and bake for 25 to 30 minutes or until top crackles and a toothpick inserted in the center comes out nearly clean.

5. Transfer to a wire rack, and cool before cutting into 16 squares. Serve from the pan, or transfer to an airtight container and store for up to 5 days.

Milk-Free Morsel

Store opened packages of sweetened flaked coconut in the refrigerator for up to 6 months.

Double-Dutch Chocolate Brownies

Intense baker's chocolate brings flavor and alleviates worry of hidden dairy in these moist, fudgy brownies, made doubly good with a dark chocolate icing.

Yield: 8 servings	
Prep time: 20 minutes	
Cook time: 40 minutes	
Serving size: 2 brownies	

3 (1-oz.) squares baker's unsweetened chocolate

⅓ cup plus 1 TB. dairy-free margarine

1 cup sugar

2 large eggs

¾ cup all-purpose flour

½ tsp. baking powder

½ tsp. salt

1 cup confectioners' sugar, or more as needed

1. Preheat the oven to 350°F. Lightly coat an 8×8-inch-square baking pan with margarine.

2. In the top of a double boiler over medium-high heat, melt 2 chocolate squares and ⅓ cup margarine, stirring occasionally.

3. Transfer mixture to a medium mixing bowl, and using an electric mixer on medium speed, beat in sugar and eggs.

4. In another bowl, whisk together flour, baking powder, and salt. Stir flour mixture into wet mixture.

5. Spread batter into the prepared pan, and bake for 30 to 35 minutes or until top crackles and a toothpick inserted in center comes out almost clean. Transfer to a wire rack to cool.

6. Make icing by melting together remaining 1 tablespoon margarine and remaining 1 chocolate square in the top of a double boiler. Allow to cool for 15 minutes, and whisk in confectioners' sugar, adding more sugar as necessary to make icing spreadable.

7. When brownies have cooled completely, spread icing evenly on top. Cut into 16 squares, and serve from the pan or remove and store in an airtight container for up to 4 days.

Milk-Free Morsel

For impromptu dairy-free baking with chocolate, keeping unsweetened cocoa powder and unsweetened baker's chocolate on hand is always a good idea.

Peanut Butter Brownies

Vegetable oil and peanut butter replace the usual butter in these amazing brownies, flavored with dark cocoa powder and a touch of vanilla.

¼ **cup vegetable oil**	¾ **cup all-purpose flour**
1 cup sugar	¼ **cup cocoa powder**
3 TB. creamy peanut butter	½ **tsp. baking powder**
2 large eggs	¼ **tsp. salt**
1 tsp. vanilla extract	

Yield: 8 servings

Prep time: 20 minutes
Cook time: 25 to 35 minutes
Serving size: 2 brownies

1. Preheat the oven to 350°F. Lightly coat an 8×8-inch-square baking pan with margarine.

2. In a medium bowl, and using an electric mixer on medium speed, beat vegetable oil and sugar. Add peanut butter, eggs, and vanilla extract, and beat until smooth.

3. In another bowl, whisk together flour, cocoa powder, baking powder, and salt. Add flour mixture to wet mixture in 2 batches, stirring well to combine after each addition.

4. Spread batter into the prepared pan, and bake for 25 to 35 minutes or until top crackles and a toothpick inserted in the center is nearly clean.

5. Transfer to a wire rack to cool, cut into 16 squares, and serve from the pan or transfer to an airtight container and store for up to 5 days.

 Milk-Free Morsel

For added texture, consider using crunchy-style peanut butter for brownie and cookie baking. Refrain from using natural-style peanut butter when baking, however, as its tendency to separate may alter the recipe.

Carrot Snack Cake with "Cream Cheese" Frosting

Perfect for daytime snacking, this favorite standby dotted with sweet pineapple and raisins gets a super-creamy frosting from handy, dairy-free ingredients.

Yield: 9 servings

Prep time: 20 minutes

Cook time: 30 to 40 minutes

Serving size: 1 (3-inch) square

---

2 large eggs

¾ cup vegetable oil

½ cup sugar

½ tsp. vanilla extract

1 cup all-purpose flour

1 tsp. baking soda

1 tsp. ground cinnamon

½ tsp. salt

1 cup grated carrots

⅓ cup chopped fresh or canned crushed pineapple

⅓ cup dark seedless raisins

½ (4-oz.) pkg. dairy-free cream cheese

2 tsp. soy creamer

1 tsp. lemon juice

1 cup confectioners' sugar, or more as needed

1. Preheat the oven to 350°F. Lightly coat a 9-inch-square baking pan with dairy-free margarine and flour.

2. In a medium bowl, and using an electric mixer on medium speed, beat eggs, vegetable oil, sugar, and vanilla extract for 2 minutes.

3. In another bowl, whisk together flour, baking soda, cinnamon, and salt. Add flour mixture to wet mixture in 2 batches, beating well after each addition.

4. Stir in carrots, pineapple, and raisins.

5. Pour into the prepared pan, and bake in the middle of the oven for 30 to 40 minutes or until a toothpick inserted in the middle comes out clean. Let cool completely in the pan on a wire rack.

6. In a medium bowl, and using an electric mixer on medium-high speed, beat cream cheese, soy creamer, lemon juice, and confectioners' sugar. Add more confectioners' sugar if necessary to make frosting spreadable.

7. When cake is cool, spread frosting over top, and serve from the pan. Store covered and refrigerated for up to 4 days.

Free Fact

Carrots have been used in baking since medieval times, when sweeteners were hard to come by. Their high sugar content, almost as high as beet sugar, made plain baked goods more dessertlike.

Italian Olive Oil Semolina Cake

This traditional Italian cake, naturally free of butter, gets its unique flavor from fruity olive oil and lemon zest and is particularly good when served drizzled with honey.

1 cup sugar	1 cup all-purpose flour
3 large eggs	½ cup *semolina* flour
2 tsp. lemon zest	2½ tsp. baking powder
¼ cup soy or almond milk	½ tsp. salt
¾ cup olive oil	Confectioners' sugar

Yield: 1 (8-inch) round cake

Prep time: 15 minutes

Cook time: 25 to 35 minutes

Serving size: ⅙ cake

1. Preheat the oven to 350°F. Lightly oil an 8-inch-round cake pan.

2. In a medium bowl, and using an electric mixer on medium speed, beat sugar and eggs for about 3 minutes or until pale and smooth. Beat in lemon zest and soy milk.

3. Slowly pour in olive oil while continuing to beat on medium speed.

4. In another bowl, whisk together all-purpose flour, semolina flour, baking powder, and salt. Add flour mixture to wet mixture, and stir just to blend.

5. Pour into the prepared pan, and bake in the middle of the oven for 30 to 40 minutes or until a toothpick inserted in the middle comes out clean.

6. Transfer to a wire rack to cool for 15 minutes, remove cake from the pan, and place on a cake platter to cool completely. Dust with confectioners' sugar before serving.

Lactose Lingo

Semolina is the coarsely ground endosperm of durum wheat used in pasta making. When more finely milled, it resembles the consistency of flour.

Rich Almond and Poppy Seed Cake

The delicious flavor of almonds highlights this speckled cake perfect for dessert but delicious any time of day.

Yield: 1 (8- or 9-inch) cake

Prep time: 30 minutes

Cook time: 40 to 50 minutes

Serving size: ¹⁄₁₂ cake

¼ cup poppy seeds

¼ cup vanilla almond milk

¼ cup (1 stick) dairy-free margarine, softened

½ cup sugar

¼ cup vegetable oil

2 tsp. almond extract

1½ cups all-purpose flour

1 TB. baking powder

5 large egg whites, at room temperature

Free Fact

Fluted tube pans, or Bundt pans, grew in popularity in the 1960s after a Pillsbury cook-off contest. National Bundt (Pan) Day, celebrated every November 15, was established shortly after.

1. Preheat the oven to 350°F. Generously coat an 8- or 9-inch fluted tube pan with dairy-free margarine and flour.

2. In a small saucepan over medium-high heat, combine poppy seeds and almond milk, and bring to a boil, stirring often. Reduce heat to low, and simmer for 5 minutes. Remove from heat, cover, and set aside to cool.

3. In a medium bowl, and using an electric mixer on medium speed, beat margarine and sugar until light and fluffy. Add vegetable oil and almond extract, and continue to beat for 1 minute or until well combined.

4. Add poppy seeds and almond milk mixture, and beat for 1 or 2 minutes or until combined. Add flour and baking powder, and continue beating for about 2 minutes or until smooth.

5. In another bowl, and with clean beaters in the mixer on high speed, beat egg whites for 2 to 3 minutes or until soft peaks form. Gently fold into poppy seed batter using a rubber spatula.

6. Evenly spoon batter into the prepared pan, and bake in the middle of the oven for 40 to 50 minutes or until edges begin to pull away from the pan and a toothpick inserted in the center comes out clean.

7. Transfer to a wire rack, and allow to cool completely before inverting onto a cake platter. Keep covered at room temperature for up to 5 days.

Angel Food Cupcakes

Light and heavenly, these cupcakes flavored with vanilla bean are perfect when a little something sweet is in order.

10 large egg whites, at room temperature

½ tsp. salt

Seeds from 1 vanilla bean

1 tsp. cream of tartar

¾ cup sugar

1 cup cake flour

½ cup confectioners' sugar

Yield: 9 servings
Prep time: 30 minutes
Cook time: 13 to 15 minutes
Serving size: 2 cupcakes

1. Preheat the oven to 325°F. Line 1½ standard muffin tins with paper or foil cupcake liners (9 cupcakes).

2. In a large bowl, combine egg whites, salt, vanilla bean seeds, and cream of tartar. Using an electric mixer on high speed, beat for 1 or 2 minutes or until soft peaks form. Beat in sugar a little at a time until whites are glossy and form firm peaks.

3. In a small bowl, whisk together cake flour and confectioners' sugar. Using a sifter or fine sieve, dust flour mixture into egg white mixture in 2 batches, folding gently each time to combine.

4. Spoon batter into the prepared cups about ⅔ full, and bake in the middle of the oven for 13 to 15 minutes or until tops are golden and a toothpick inserted in the center comes out clean.

5. Transfer cupcakes to a wire rack to cool before serving. Keep in an airtight container for up to 4 days.

Milk-Free Morsel

To collect seeds from a vanilla bean, use a sharp knife to cut the bean in half lengthwise, open the bean gently, and use the back of the knife to scrape out the seeds.

Deep-Chocolate-Glazed Cupcakes

Rich and deliciously decadent, these cupcakes topped with a bittersweet chocolate glaze will satisfy anyone's chocolate fantasy.

Yield: 24 cupcakes	
Prep time: 30 minutes	
Cook time: 30 minutes	
Serving size: 1 or 2 cupcakes	

½ cup soy milk

1 tsp. cider vinegar

2 (1-oz.) squares baker's unsweetened chocolate

½ cup plus 2 TB. dairy-free margarine

1 cup boiling water

2 cups sugar

2 cups all-purpose flour

1½ tsp. baking soda

½ tsp. salt

2 large eggs, slightly beaten

6 oz. dairy-free bittersweet chocolate, roughly chopped

1 TB. light corn syrup

1. Preheat the oven to 350°F. Line 2 standard muffin tins with paper or foil cupcake liners (24 cupcakes).

2. In a small bowl, combine soy milk and vinegar. Set aside.

3. In the top of a double boiler set over medium-high heat, melt unsweetened chocolate squares and ½ cup margarine, stirring occasionally. Remove from heat, and stir in boiling water. Set aside.

4. Place sugar in a large bowl, and using an electric mixer on medium speed, beat in chocolate mixture.

5. In another bowl, whisk together flour, baking soda, and salt. Add flour mixture to wet mixture in 2 batches, beating well to combine. Add eggs and reserved soy milk mixture, and beat for 1 more minute.

6. Divide batter among muffin cups, and bake in the middle of the oven for 20 to 25 minutes or until a toothpick inserted in the center comes out clean. Transfer to a wire rack to cool.

7. Meanwhile, in a small saucepan over low heat, melt bittersweet chocolate, remaining 2 tablespoons margarine, and corn syrup, whisking often. Remove from heat, and set aside for 10 minutes.

8. Pour a little glaze on top of each cupcake, and allow to set for 30 minutes before serving.

Milk-Free Morsel

Keep leftover chocolate glaze in the refrigerator for up to 2 weeks. Remelt it for topping on cakes, fruit, or dairy-free ice cream by microwaving at medium strength for 10-second intervals or in a saucepan over low heat.

Chapter 18

Puddings, Pies, and Frozen Treats

In This Chapter

◆ Creamy dairy-free puddings

◆ Pie making as easy as … pie!

◆ Cool ice creams and other frozen dairy-free delights

If puddings have been off-limits from your dairy-free diet, it's time to grab your spoon and dig in to the unbelievably delicious puddings featured in this chapter. They're all super-creamy and flavor-packed, and you'll have a hard time deciding which to make first.

But that's not all. If pie's your thing, you've come to the right place. This chapter offers dairy-free piecrusts and fillings you'll want to use again and again. And for nights when fruit is on the dessert menu, a classic apple crisp or fresh strawberry pie might be just the thing.

Finally, when it comes to good old-fashioned ice cream, many a dairy-free eater has found disappointment in substitutes that pale to the original. Fortunately, that will be behind you when you taste the outstanding results of the frozen "ice creams" in this chapter. So grab your ice-cream maker!

Creamy Dreamy Rice Pudding

You'll soon find yourself whipping up batches of this easy, rich, and creamy rice pudding, lightly flavored with cinnamon, vanilla, and banana, quite often.

Yield: 6 servings	
Prep time: 1 hour, 15 minutes	
Cook time: 30 minutes	
Serving size: about ½ cup	

1 TB. cornstarch

⅓ cup vanilla soy creamer

1 medium, ripe banana

1 cup dry white *basmati rice*, cooked according to pkg. directions (about 3 cups cooked)

3 cups vanilla rice milk

½ cup light brown sugar, firmly packed

½ tsp. ground cinnamon, plus more for sprinkling

1. In a blender, purée cornstarch, vanilla soy creamer, and banana for about 1 minute or until smooth. Set aside.

2. In a large saucepan over medium-low heat, combine warm cooked rice, vanilla rice milk, light brown sugar, and cinnamon, and stir well to combine. Bring to a low simmer, and cook, stirring often, for 10 minutes. Add banana mixture, and cook for 10 more minutes as it thickens, stirring frequently.

3. Transfer to a large bowl, cover the surface with plastic wrap, and refrigerate for about 1 hour or until cold. Sprinkle with cinnamon before serving.

Lactose Lingo

Basmati rice is a delicate, fragrant rice often used in Indian cooking. It's available at most supermarkets.

Tapioca Pudding Parfait

Layers of creamy tapioca combine with sweet preserves in this impressive yet easy pudding dessert that's completely dairy free.

½ cup small-pearl tapioca
(not instant)

1½ cups soy milk

1½ cups rice milk

½ tsp. salt

½ cup sugar

2 large eggs, beaten

½ tsp. vanilla extract

1½ cups raspberry or other
fruit preserves

4 oz. fresh raspberries (about
½ cup)

Yield: 6 servings
Prep time: 1 hour, 15 minutes
Cook time: 12 minutes
Serving size: 1 parfait

1. In a medium saucepan over medium heat, combine tapioca, soy milk, rice milk, and salt. Bring to a simmer, stirring occasionally, and cook for 5 minutes. Remove from heat and stir in sugar.

2. Spoon a little tapioca mixture into beaten eggs, and whisk egg mixture to the saucepan. Cook over low heat, stirring often, for about 8 minutes or until well thickened.

3. Stir in vanilla extract, remove from heat, and set aside to cool slightly.

4. To make parfaits, alternate spooning a little tapioca, followed by a spoonful of raspberry preserves, into 6 fluted glasses to create 4 or 5 layers. Top with raspberries, and refrigerate for at least 1 hour before serving.

Free Fact

Tapioca comes from the cassava or yucca plant and is not, as sometimes reported, an animal protein derivative.

Unbelievable Chocolate Pudding

Thanks to a double dose of chocolate, you won't believe how intense the flavor is and how rich the consistency is in this pudding.

Yield: *4 servings*
Prep time: 1 hour, 20 minutes
Cook time: 10 minutes
Serving size: about ⅔ cup

½ **cup cocoa powder**

6 TB. cornstarch

⅓ **cup sugar**

Pinch salt

3 cups chocolate soy milk

1 tsp. vanilla extract

1. In a medium saucepan, whisk together cocoa powder, cornstarch, sugar, and salt. Gradually whisk in chocolate soy milk until smooth.

2. Cook, whisking constantly, over medium heat for about 10 minutes or until thickened and bubbly. Remove from heat, and stir in vanilla extract.

3. Divide among 4 pudding cups, cover the surface with plastic wrap, and allow to cool for 10 minutes before transferring to the refrigerator to cool for about 1 hour.

Free Fact

Vanilla is always added to chocolate creations because it brings out the best in chocolate ingredients by pushing the flavor forward.

Best-Ever Lemon Meringue Pie

A flaky piecrust, intense lemon filling, and a perfect glossy meringue come together in this hands-down best summer pie favorite.

Yield: 1 (9-inch) pie	
Prep time: 30 minutes	
Cook time: 30 minutes	
Serving size: ⅛ pie	

1 cup all-purpose flour, plus more for rolling

½ tsp. salt

⅓ cup dairy-free margarine or vegetable shortening

2 TB. cold water

1½ cups plus 6 TB. sugar

⅓ cup cornstarch

1½ cups water

3 large egg yolks, beaten

3 TB. dairy-free margarine

¼ cup lemon juice

1½ TB. grated lemon zest

3 large egg whites

¼ tsp. cream of tartar

1. Preheat the oven to 425°F.

2. In a medium bowl, combine flour and salt. Add ⅓ cup margarine, and using a fork or pastry blender, mix with flour to a sandy consistency. Add cold water, and gather dough into a ball.

3. Turn out dough onto a work surface, and roll out to fit a 9-inch pie pan, using extra flour as necessary to keep dough from sticking. Transfer to the pie pan, crimp edges, and bake for 6 to 8 minutes or until lightly browned. Remove from the oven and set aside.

4. In a medium saucepan over medium heat, whisk together 1½ cups sugar, cornstarch, and water. Bring to a boil, and cook, stirring constantly, for about 5 minutes or until thickened. Continue to cook for 1 more minute.

5. Add a small amount of cornstarch mixture to beaten eggs, stirring well. Whisk egg mixture to the saucepan, and cook, stirring, for 1 more minute.

6. Remove from heat; stir in remaining 3 tablespoons margarine, lemon juice, and lemon rind; and pour into baked pie shell.

7. In a medium bowl, and using an electric mixer on high speed, beat egg whites and cream of tartar until soft peaks form. Gradually add remaining 6 tablespoons sugar, and continue beating for 2 minutes or until firm, glossy peaks form.

8. Spoon meringue on top of lemon filling, spreading evenly to cover all the way to crust edges and making peaks with the back of a spoon. Bake for 6 to 8 minutes or until peaks turn golden brown and meringue is set. Cool completely before serving.

Free Fact

Cream of tartar contains no cream or dairy in any form. It is simply the salt by-product of tartaric acid, often used to stabilize egg whites or prevent food discoloration.

Summer Strawberry Pie with Graham Cracker Crust

This delicious and practically no-bake pie features succulent ripe strawberries and a dairy-free crust that's sweet and crisp.

1½ cups dairy-free graham cracker crumbs

5 TB. sugar

1 TB. all-purpose flour

4 TB. dairy-free margarine, melted

2½ cups fresh strawberries, washed, stems removed, and halved

1¼ cups cranberry-strawberry juice

4 TB. cornstarch

Yield: 1 (9-inch) pie		
Prep time: 30 minutes		
Cook time: 15 minutes		
Serving size: ⅛ pie		

1. Preheat the oven to 350°F. Lightly coat a 9-inch pie pan with vegetable oil.

2. In a medium bowl, stir together graham cracker crumbs, 3 tablespoons sugar, flour, and melted margarine until well combined. Transfer to the pie pan, and press evenly up the sides and on the bottom. Bake for 10 to 12 minutes or until set and lightly golden. Remove from the oven, and set aside to cool.

3. In a medium bowl, add strawberries and sprinkle remaining 2 tablespoons sugar over top, tossing well to coat. Set aside.

4. In a medium saucepan over medium heat, whisk together cranberry-strawberry juice and cornstarch until dissolved. Bring to a low boil, whisking constantly, and cook for 2 minutes or until thickened. Boil for 1 more minute, and remove from heat.

5. Add thickened juice to strawberries, and stir gently with a rubber spatula to coat. Transfer to baked piecrust, and spread out evenly. Chill in the refrigerator for 2 hours before serving.

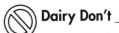 **Dairy Don't**

Be careful of readymade piecrusts because they often contain milk derivatives even if they don't contain butter.

Coconut Custard Pie with Macadamia Nut Crust

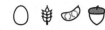

A rich and creamy coconut filling highlights this super-tasty pie with a tropical, nutty-flavored crust.

Yield: 1 (9-inch) pie	
Prep time: 3 hours, 30 minutes	
Cook time: 30 minutes	
Serving size: ⅛ pie	

5 oz. macadamia nuts, toasted and ground

½ cup panko breadcrumbs

1¼ cup sugar

2 TB. plus ½ cup all-purpose flour

3 TB. dairy-free margarine, melted

¼ tsp. salt

3 cups unsweetened coconut milk

3 large egg yolks, beaten

2 TB. dairy-free margarine

1½ tsp. vanilla extract

1 cup sweetened flaked coconut

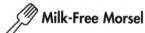

Milk-Free Morsel

To toast macadamia nuts or any other type of nut, arrange in a single layer on a rimmed baking sheet and bake in a 350°F oven for about 10 minutes, occasionally shaking the pan to brown evenly. If using them for a crust, allow them to cool before grinding in a food processor.

1. Preheat the oven to 375°F.

2. In a medium bowl, combine ground macadamia nuts, panko breadcrumbs, ¼ cup sugar, 2 tablespoons flour, and melted margarine, stirring well to combine. Transfer to 9-inch pie pan, and press evenly up the sides and on the bottom. Bake for about 20 minutes or until lightly golden. Remove from the oven, and set aside.

3. In a medium saucepan over medium heat, combine remaining 1 cup sugar, remaining ½ cup flour, and salt. Gradually stir in coconut milk, and cook, stirring, for 1 or 2 minutes or until thick and bubbly. Remove from heat, and spoon a little hot mixture into eggs, stirring well.

4. Add egg mixture to the saucepan, and continue to cook at a gentle boil for 2 minutes.

5. Remove from heat, and stir in 2 tablespoons margarine, vanilla extract, and coconut. Pour into baked crust, and allow to cool for 10 minutes.

6. Cover with plastic wrap, and cool completely in the refrigerator for about 3 hours before serving.

Caramel-Apple Crisp

This delectable favorite features sweet apples and a crispy oat topping with hints of sugar and nutmeg. A quick caramel drizzle takes it to even greater heights.

4 large firm apples, such as Golden Delicious

¾ cup light brown sugar, firmly packed

½ cup all-purpose flour

½ cup old-fashioned rolled oats

⅓ cup dairy-free margarine, softened

1 tsp. ground cinnamon

¼ tsp. ground nutmeg

½ cup sugar

¼ cup water

3 TB. dairy-free margarine

¼ cup soy creamer

Yield: 4 servings
Prep time: 20 minutes
Cook time: 45 minutes
Serving size: 1 cup

1. Preheat the oven to 375°F. Lightly coat an 8-inch-square baking pan with dairy-free margarine.

2. Peel and core apples, and slice into ½-inch-thick pieces. Spread evenly in the prepared pan.

3. In a medium bowl, stir together brown sugar, flour, oats, softened margarine, cinnamon, and nutmeg. Sprinkle evenly over apples. Bake for about 30 minutes or until topping is golden and apples are fork-tender.

4. In a medium saucepan over medium heat, combine sugar and water. Cook, stirring occasionally, for about 10 minutes or until caramel begins to brown. Remove from heat, and whisk in 3 tablespoons margarine. Slowly whisk in soy creamer, and continue whisking until smooth.

5. Drizzle caramel over top of baked apple crisp, and allow to set for 10 minutes before serving.

Free Fact

Yellow or Golden Delicious apples are not actually related to the Red Delicious apple, but they were so named because of their similar eating and cooking qualities.

Vanilla Bean Ice Cream

Super creamy with flecks of delicious vanilla bean, you'll be amazed how perfect this dairy-free ice cream can be.

Yield: 2 cups

Prep time: 10 minutes

Cook time: 12 minutes

Serving size: ½ cup

1½ cups soy creamer

½ cup soy milk

Seeds from 1 vanilla bean

½ cup sugar

4 large egg yolks, at room temperature

1. In a medium saucepan over medium heat, combine soy creamer, soy milk, and vanilla bean seeds. Bring to a simmer, whisking occasionally; remove from heat; and set aside.

2. In a medium mixing bowl, and using an electric mixer on medium speed, beat sugar and egg yolks for 1 or 2 minutes or until pale ribbons form when you lift the beaters.

3. Slowly add ½ of milk mixture to egg mixture, whisking well. Pour into remaining milk in the saucepan, and cook over medium-low heat, stirring constantly, for 2 or 3 minutes or until mixture thickens somewhat and coats the back of a spoon.

4. Immediately pour through a fine sieve into a bowl, cover top with plastic wrap, and cool for 10 minutes. Refrigerate for at least 1 hour or until very cold.

5. Pour into an ice-cream maker and, following the manufacturer's instructions, churn until thick and creamy. Transfer to an airtight container, and keep frozen for up to 5 days.

⊘ Dairy Don't

Well-intentioned hosts may serve lactose-free ice cream to dairy-free eaters, not realizing it actually contains dairy, so be mindful when eating out.

Peachy Almond Ice Cream

The complementary flavors of fresh peaches and delicious almond highlight this creamy frozen treat.

1 cup vanilla almond milk

1 cup soy creamer

½ tsp. almond extract

¼ cup sugar

2 medium ripe peaches, peeled, seed removed, and diced

2 TB. sliced almonds

Yield: 2 cups
Prep time: 20 minutes
Cook time: 10 minutes
Serving size: ½ cup

1. In a medium saucepan over medium heat, combine vanilla almond milk, soy creamer, almond extract, and sugar. Cook, whisking occasionally, for 3 to 5 minutes or until sugar has dissolved and mixture begins to bubble.

2. Add peaches and cook for 1 more minute.

3. Remove from heat, transfer mixture to a bowl, cover the surface, and allow to cool for 10 minutes. Refrigerate for at least 1 hour or until very cold.

4. Stir in sliced almonds.

5. Pour into an ice-cream maker and, following the manufacturer's instructions, churn until thick and creamy. Transfer to an airtight container, and store in the freezer for up to 5 days.

Free Fact

Peaches are the second-largest commercially grown fruit crop in the United States, after apples.

Frozen Holiday Egg Nog

You'll dazzle holiday guests with this delightful dessert featuring the rich flavor of egg nog and a dollop of cream, all amazingly dairy-free!

Yield: 2 cups	
Prep time: 20 minutes	
Cook time: 1½ hour	
Serving size: ½ cup	

2 cups soy "egg nog"

2 TB. soy milk

1 TB. cornstarch

½ cup coconut cream, chilled

2 TB. confectioners' sugar

Dash ground nutmeg

1. Heat egg nog in a medium saucepan over medium heat, whisking occasionally, until it just begins to boil.

2. In a small bowl stir together soy milk and cornstarch until smooth. While whisking the egg nog, pour in the cornstarch mixture and continue whisking for 2 minutes while mixture cooks at a low boil and thickens.

3. Transfer the mixture to a bowl, cover and refrigerate for at least 1 hour or until well chilled.

4. Pour the mixture into an ice cream maker and, following manufacturer's directions, churn until cold and thickened. Transfer to the freezer until ready to serve.

5. When ready to compose dessert, combine coconut cream and confectioners' sugar in a medium bowl and beat with an electric mixer on high until soft peaks form.

6. To serve, scoop the frozen egg nog into 4 punch glasses and smooth the top with the back of a spoon. Top each with a dollop of the whipped coconut cream and a dash of nutmeg.

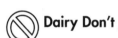

Dairy Don't

Holiday party buffet tables are often rife with food containing dairy. Always ask about the ingredients before dishing up.

Toasted Coconut Sorbet

Full of sweet coconut flavor and with a creamy texture, this sorbet is refreshing on a hot summer day.

2 cups sweetened coconut cream	1 TB. water
1 tsp. lemon juice	½ cup toasted shredded coconut

Yield: 2 cups
Prep time: 20 minutes
Serving size: ½ cup

1. In a medium bowl, whisk together coconut milk, lemon juice, and water. Refrigerate for at least 1 hour or until very cold.

2. Stir in toasted coconut.

3. Pour into an ice-cream maker and, following the manufacturer's instructions, churn until thick and creamy. Transfer to an airtight container, and store in the freezer for up to 1 week.

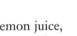 **Milk-Free Morsel**

Toast sweetened or unsweetened shredded coconut in a large, nonstick pan over medium heat, stirring often, for 3 or 4 minutes or until golden.

Dark Chocolate Sorbet

Intense dark chocolate flavor is the only way to describe this decadent frozen treat all chocolate lovers will flip over.

Yield: 2 cups
Prep time: 10 minutes
Cook time: 5 minutes
Serving size: ½ cup

1 cup sugar

½ cup cocoa powder

2 cups water

½ cup finely chopped dairy-free bittersweet chocolate

1. In a medium saucepan over medium heat, whisk sugar and cocoa powder. Slowly add water, whisking to combine well. Bring to a low boil, whisking often, and cook for 1 minute.

2. Transfer to a bowl, cover with plastic wrap, and allow to cool for 10 minutes. Refrigerate for at least 1½ hours or until very cold.

3. Stir in chopped chocolate.

4. Pour into an ice-cream maker and, following the manufacturer's instructions, churn until thick and creamy. Transfer to an airtight container, and store in the freezer for up to 1 week.

 Milk-Free Morsel

When chopping blocks of chocolate, use a chilled plastic board to help keep the chocolate cool and, therefore, easier to cut. Also always chop *away* from you on a 45-degree angle.

Frozen Strawberry Soufflé

Light and airy, with the delicious flavor of sweet strawberries, this frozen dessert will make a big splash when served to family and friends.

2 TB. meringue powder

¼ **cup cold water**

⅓ **cup sugar**

1 tsp. vanilla extract

½ **cup light corn syrup**

2 cups frozen strawberries in light syrup

1 tsp. lemon juice

¼ **cup grated dairy-free bittersweet chocolate**

Yield: 8 servings	
Prep time: 55 minutes	
Serving size: ½ cup	

1. In a medium bowl, and with an electric mixer on high speed, beat meringue powder and water for about 1 minute or until soft peaks form.

2. Gradually beat in sugar for about 2 minutes or until stiff peaks form. Beat in vanilla extract. Slowly pour corn syrup into meringue mixture while beating on high speed. Beat for about 3 more minutes or until frosting is thick and spreadable. Refrigerate for 30 minutes.

3. Fold a piece of parchment paper 20 inches long in half lengthwise to form a long strip. Wrap around a 1½-quart round casserole or soufflé dish. Secure with tape, and leave at least 4 inches of paper above the rim of the casserole.

4. In a blender, purée strawberries and syrup for about 1 minute or until smooth. Strain through a fine sieve into a large bowl. Stir in lemon juice.

5. A little at a time, stir marshmallow frosting into strawberry purée, without overmixing. Transfer to the prepared dish, allowing mixture to come up the sides of the paper wrapping, and smooth over the top. Cover the top surface with plastic wrap, and freeze for at least 3 hours or overnight.

6. Just before serving and slicing, remove the paper wrap and sprinkle grated chocolate on top. Keep any leftovers well wrapped in the freezer.

 Dairy Don't

Frozen dessert soufflés (as well as nonfrozen versions) are usually made with milk or cream, so be sure to ask when dining out.

Pink Lemonade Ice

Like a classic Italian ice, this pretty pink, sweet-yet-tart frozen delight will refresh and satisfy on the hottest of days.

Yield: 2 cups
Prep time: 45 minutes
Serving size: ½ cup

½ cup fresh lemon juice

⅔ cup *superfine sugar*

½ cup crushed ice

2 cups water

1 tsp. *grenadine*

1. In a blender, purée lemon juice, sugar, ice, water, and grenadine for about 1 minute or until smooth.

2. Pour into 4 freezable custard or paper cups, and cover the surface with plastic wrap. Freeze for at least 30 minutes or until solid, and serve.

Lactose Lingo

Grenadine is a sweet pomegranate-based syrup often used to flavor and color cocktails. **Superfine sugar,** also used frequently in cocktails, dissolves completely in liquid without heating unlike regular sugar.

Glossary

al dente   Italian for "against the teeth." Refers to pasta or rice that's neither soft nor hard, but just slightly firm against the teeth.

all-purpose flour   Flour that contains only the inner part of the wheat grain. Usable for all purposes, from cakes to gravies.

allspice   Named for its flavor echoes of several spices (cinnamon, cloves, nutmeg), allspice is used in many desserts and in rich marinades and stews.

almonds   Mild, sweet, and crunchy nuts that combine nicely with creamy and sweet food items.

anaphylaxis   A serious allergic reaction—possibly fatal—that comes on quickly after milk is ingested.

anchovies (also **sardines**)   Tiny, flavorful preserved fish that typically come in cans. Anchovies are a traditional garnish for Caesar salad, the dressing of which contains anchovy paste.

andouille sausage   A sausage made with highly seasoned pork chitterlings and tripe, and a standard component of many Cajun dishes.

antipasto   A classic Italian-style appetizer, usually served together as one course or plate, including an assortment of prepared meats, cheeses, and vegetables such as prosciutto, capicolla, mozzarella, mushrooms, and olives.

arborio rice   A plump Italian rice used, among other purposes, for risotto.

artichoke hearts   The center part of the artichoke flower, often found canned in grocery stores.

arugula   A spicy-peppery garden plant with leaves that resemble a dandelion and have a distinctive—and very sharp—flavor.

au gratin   The quick broiling of a dish before serving, to brown the top ingredients. When used in a recipe name, the term often implies cheese and a creamy sauce.

bake   To cook in a dry oven. Dry-heat cooking often results in a crisping of the exterior of the food being cooked. Moist-heat cooking, through methods such as steaming and poaching, brings a much different, moist quality to the food.

balsamic vinegar   Vinegar produced primarily in Italy from a specific type of grape and aged in wood barrels. It is heavier, darker, and sweeter than most vinegars.

bamboo shoots   Crunchy, tasty white parts of the growing bamboo plant, often purchased canned.

barbecue   To quick-cook over high heat, or to cook something long and slow in a rich liquid (barbecue sauce).

basil   A flavorful, almost sweet, resinous herb delicious with tomatoes and used in all kinds of Italian or Mediterranean-style dishes.

basmati rice   A delicate, fragrant rice often used in Indian cooking.

baste   To keep foods moist during cooking by spooning, brushing, or drizzling with a liquid.

beat   To quickly mix substances.

black pepper   A biting and pungent seasoning, freshly ground pepper is a must for many dishes and adds an extra level of flavor and taste.

blackening   To cook something quickly in a very hot skillet over high heat, usually with a seasoning mixture. Cajun cooking makes frequent use of blackening.

blanch   To place a food in boiling water for about 1 minute (or less) to partially cook the exterior, and then submerge in or rinse with cool water to halt the cooking.

blend   To completely mix something, usually with a blender or food processor, more slowly than beating.

blue cheese   A blue-veined cheese that crumbles easily and has a somewhat soft texture, usually sold in a block. The color is from a flavorful, edible mold that is often added or injected into the cheese.

boil   To heat a liquid to a point where water is forced to turn into steam, causing the liquid to bubble. To boil something is to insert it into boiling water. In a rapid boil, a lot of bubbles form on the surface of the liquid.

bok choy (also **Chinese cabbage**)   A member of the cabbage family, with thick stems, crisp texture, and fresh flavor. It's perfect for stir-frying.

bouillon   Dried essence of stock from chicken, beef, vegetable, or other ingredients. This is a popular starting ingredient for soups, as it adds flavor (and often a lot of salt).

braise   To cook with the introduction of some liquid, usually over an extended period of time.

breadcrumbs   Tiny pieces of crumbled dry bread, often used for topping or coating.

brine   A highly salted, often seasoned, liquid used to flavor and preserve foods. To brine a food is to soak or preserve it by submerging it in brine. The salt in the brine penetrates the fibers of the meat and makes it moist and tender.

broil   To cook in a dry oven under the overhead high-heat element.

broth   *See* stock.

brown   To cook in a skillet, turning, until the food's surface is seared and brown in color, to lock in the juices.

brown rice   Whole-grain rice, including the germ, with a characteristic pale brown or tan color; more nutritious and flavorful than white rice.

bruschetta (or **crostini**)   Slices of toasted or grilled bread with garlic and olive oil, often with other toppings.

bulgur   A wheat kernel that has been steamed, dried, and crushed, sold in fine and coarse textures.

Cajun cooking   A style of cooking that combines French and Southern characteristics and includes many highly seasoned stews and meats.

canapés   Bite-size hors d'oeuvres usually served on a small piece of bread or toast.

capers   Flavorful buds of a Mediterranean plant, ranging in size from *nonpareil* (about the size of a small pea) to larger, grape-size caper berries produced in Spain.

caramelize   To cook sugar over low heat until it develops a sweet caramel flavor. The term is increasingly gaining use to describe cooking vegetables (especially onions) or meat in butter or oil over low heat until they soften, sweeten, and develop a caramel color.

caraway A distinctive spicy seed used for bread, pork, cheese, and cabbage dishes. It is known to reduce stomach upset, which is why it is often paired with, for example, sauerkraut.

carbohydrate A nutritional component found in starches, sugars, fruits, and vegetables that causes a rise in blood glucose levels. Carbohydrates supply energy and many important nutrients, including vitamins, minerals, and antioxidants.

cardamom An intense, sweet-smelling spice, common to Indian cooking, used in baking and coffee.

carob A tropical tree that produces long pods. The dried, baked, and powdered flesh (carob powder) is used in baking, and the fresh and dried pods are used for a variety of recipes. The flavor is sweet and reminiscent of chocolate.

casein A protein found in all dairy products, including cheese, milk, and yogurt. It's often added to many processed foods as well.

cayenne A fiery spice made from (hot) chili peppers, especially the cayenne chili, a slender, red, and very hot pepper.

celeriac Also known as celery root or knob celery, celeriac is a root vegetable with a strong flavor and taste of celery.

chili powder A seasoning blend that includes chili pepper, cumin, garlic, and oregano. Proportions vary among different versions, but they all offer a warm, rich flavor.

chilis (or **chiles**) Any one of many different "hot" peppers, ranging in intensity from the relatively mild ancho pepper to the blisteringly hot habañero.

Chinese five-spice powder A seasoning blend of cinnamon, anise, ginger, fennel, and pepper.

chipotle peppers Smoked jalapeño peppers, dark in color and almost chocolatelike in flavor.

chives A member of the onion family, chives grow in bunches of long leaves that resemble tall grass or the green tops of onions and offer a light onion flavor.

chop To cut into pieces, usually qualified by an adverb such as "*coarsely* chopped," or by a size measurement such as "chopped into $1/2$-inch pieces." "Finely chopped" is much closer to minced.

chorizo A spiced pork sausage eaten alone and as a component in many recipes.

chutney   A thick condiment often served with Indian curries, made with fruits and/or vegetables with vinegar, sugar, and spices.

cider vinegar   Vinegar produced from apple cider, popular in North America.

cilantro   A member of the parsley family and used in Mexican cooking (especially salsa) and some Asian dishes. Use in moderation, as the flavor can overwhelm. The seed of the cilantro is the spice coriander.

cinnamon   A sweet, rich, aromatic spice commonly used in baking or desserts. Cinnamon can also be used for delicious and interesting entrées.

clove   A sweet, strong, almost wintergreen-flavor spice used in baking and with meats such as ham.

coriander   A rich, warm, spicy seed used in all types of recipes, from African to South American, from entrées to desserts.

count   In terms of seafood or other foods that come in small sizes, the number of that item that compose 1 pound. For example, 31 to 40 count shrimp are large appetizer shrimp often served with cocktail sauce; 51 to 60 are much smaller.

couscous   Granular semolina (durum wheat) that is cooked and used in many Mediterranean and North African dishes.

crimini mushrooms   A relative of the white button mushroom, but brown in color and with a richer flavor. The larger, fully grown version is the portobello. *See also* portobello mushrooms.

cross-contact   Contamination by proximity of one item to another.

cross-reactivity   An allergy to one food substance may result in an allergy to another food that has similar proteins.

croutons   Chunks of bread, usually between $1/4$ and $1/2$ inch in size, sometimes seasoned and baked, broiled, or fried to a crisp texture and used in soups and salads.

crudités   Fresh vegetables served as an appetizer, often all together on one tray.

cumin   A fiery, smoky-tasting spice popular in Middle-Eastern and Indian dishes. Cumin is a seed; ground cumin seed is the most common form used in cooking.

curd   A gelatinous substance resulting from coagulated milk used to make cheese. Curd also refers to dishes of similar texture, such as dishes make with egg (lemon curd).

curing A method of preserving uncooked foods, usually meats or fish, by either salting and smoking or pickling.

curry Rich, spicy, Indian-style sauces and the dishes prepared with them. A curry uses curry powder as its base seasoning.

curry powder A ground blend of rich and flavorful spices used as a basis for curry and many other Indian-influenced dishes. Common ingredients include hot pepper, nutmeg, cumin, cinnamon, pepper, and turmeric. Some curry can also be found in paste form.

custard A cooked mixture of eggs and milk, popular as base for desserts.

dash A few drops, usually of a liquid, released by a quick shake of, for example, a bottle of hot sauce.

deglaze To scrape up the bits of meat and seasoning left in a pan or skillet after cooking. Usually this is done by adding a liquid such as wine or broth and creating a flavorful stock that can be used to create sauces.

devein To remove the dark vein from the back of a large shrimp with a sharp knife.

dice To cut into small cubes about $1/4$ inch square.

Dijon mustard Hearty, spicy mustard made in the style of the Dijon region of France.

dill An herb perfect for eggs, salmon, cheese dishes, and, of course, vegetables (pickles!).

dollop A spoonful of something creamy and thick, like sour cream or whipped cream.

double boiler A set of two pots designed to nest together, one inside the other, and provide consistent, moist heat for foods that need delicate treatment. The bottom pot holds water (not quite touching the bottom of the top pot); the top pot holds the ingredient you want to heat.

dredge To cover a piece of food with a dry substance such as flour or cornmeal.

drizzle To lightly sprinkle drops of a liquid over food, often as the finishing touch to a dish.

dry In the context of wine, a wine that contains little or no residual sugar so it's not very sweet.

emulsion A combination of liquid ingredients that do not normally mix well beaten together to create a thick liquid, such as a fat or oil with water. Creation of an emulsion must be done carefully and rapidly to ensure that particles of one ingredient are suspended in the other.

entrée The main dish in a meal. In France, however, the entrée is considered the first course.

extra-virgin olive oil *See* olive oil.

fennel In seed form, a fragrant, licorice-tasting herb. The bulbs have a much milder flavor and a celerylike crunch and are used as a vegetable in salads or cooked recipes.

fillet A piece of meat or seafood with the bones removed.

flake To break into thin sections, as with fish.

floret The flower or bud end of broccoli or cauliflower.

flour Grains ground into a meal. Wheat is perhaps the most common flour. Flour is also made from oats, rye, buckwheat, soybeans, and similar grains. *See also* all-purpose flour; cake flour; whole-wheat flour.

fold To combine a dense and light mixture with a circular action from the middle of the bowl.

frittata A skillet-cooked mixture of eggs and other ingredients that's not stirred but is cooked slowly and then either flipped or finished under the broiler.

fry *See* sauté.

garbanzo beans (or **chickpeas**) A yellow-gold, roundish bean used as the base ingredient in hummus. Chickpeas are high in fiber and low in fat.

garlic A member of the onion family, a pungent and flavorful element in many savory dishes. A garlic bulb contains multiple cloves. Each clove, when chopped, provides about 1 teaspoon garlic. Most recipes call for cloves or chopped garlic by the teaspoon.

garnish An embellishment not vital to the dish but added to enhance visual appeal.

ginger Available in fresh root or dried, ground form, ginger adds a pungent, sweet, and spicy quality to a dish.

grate To shave into tiny pieces using a sharp rasp or grater.

grenadine   A sweet pomegranate-based syrup often used to flavor and color cocktails.

grind   To reduce a large, hard substance, often a seasoning such as peppercorns, to the consistency of sand.

grits   Coarsely ground grains, usually corn.

handful   An unscientific measurement; the amount of an ingredient you can hold in your hand.

hazelnuts (also **filberts**)   A sweet nut popular in desserts and, to a lesser degree, in savory dishes.

hearts of palm   Firm, elongated, off-white cylinders from the inside of a palm tree stem tip.

herbes de Provence   A seasoning mix including basil, fennel, marjoram, rosemary, sage, and thyme, common in the south of France.

hoisin sauce   A sweet Asian condiment similar to ketchup, made with soybeans, sesame, chili peppers, and sugar.

hors d'oeuvre   French for "outside of work" (the "work" being the main meal), an hors d'oeuvre can be any dish served as a starter before the meal.

horseradish   A sharp, spicy root that forms the flavor base in many condiments, from cocktail sauce to sharp mustards. Prepared horseradish contains vinegar and oil, among other ingredients. Use pure horseradish much more sparingly than the prepared version, or try cutting it with sour cream.

hummus   A thick, Middle Eastern spread made of puréed garbanzo beans, lemon juice, olive oil, garlic, and often tahini (sesame seed paste).

infusion   A liquid in which flavorful ingredients such as herbs have been soaked or steeped to extract that flavor into the liquid.

Italian seasoning   A blend of dried herbs, including basil, oregano, rosemary, and thyme.

julienne   A French word meaning "to slice into very thin pieces."

kalamata olives   Traditionally from Greece, these medium-small long black olives have a smoky, rich flavor.

Key limes   Very small limes grown primarily in Florida, known for their tart taste.

knead   To work dough to make it pliable so it holds gas bubbles as it bakes. Kneading is fundamental in the process of making yeast breads.

kosher salt   A coarse-grained salt made without any additives or iodine.

lactase   The enzyme required to digest lactose.

lactose   The sugar present in milk.

lactose intolerance   An inability to properly digest the sugar in milk.

lentils   Tiny lens-shape pulses used in European, Middle Eastern, and Indian cuisines.

macerate   To mix sugar or another sweetener with fruit. The fruit softens, and its juice is released to mix with the sweetener.

marinate   To soak meat, seafood, or other food in a seasoned sauce, called a marinade, which is high in acid content. The acids break down the muscle of the meat, making it tender and adding flavor.

marjoram   A sweet herb, a cousin of and similar to oregano, popular in Greek, Spanish, and Italian dishes.

marshmallow   A confection made from sugar or corn syrup, water, gelatin, and flavorings.

mascarpone   A thick, creamy, spreadable cheese, traditionally from Italy.

meld   To allow flavors to blend and spread over time. Melding is often why recipes call for overnight refrigeration and is also why some dishes taste better as leftovers.

meringue powder   A baking ingredient made of dehydrated egg whites.

meringue   A baked mixture of sugar and beaten egg whites, often used as a dessert topping.

mesclun   Mixed salad greens, usually containing lettuce and assorted greens such as arugula, cress, endive, and others.

milk allergy   An immune system reaction to contact with milk proteins, resulting in sudden, potentially life-threatening symptoms, or chronic symptoms.

mince   To cut into very small pieces smaller than diced pieces, about $1/8$ inch or smaller.

miso   A fermented, flavorful soybean paste, key in many Japanese dishes.

mold   A decorative, shaped metal pan in which contents, such as mousse or gelatin, set up and take the shape of the pan.

mull (or **mulled**)   To heat a liquid with the addition of spices and sometimes sweeteners.

nutmeg   A sweet, fragrant, musky spice used primarily in baking.

nutritional yeast flakes   A deactivated yeast product high in protein and B vitamins, with a nutty and cheesy flavor.

oat milk   Made from oat groats, water, and sometimes other grains or beans. It's a good dairy-free substitute for reduced-fat or skim milk, as it's lightly textured and mildly flavored.

Old Bay Seasoning   A classic blend of herbs and spices created in the 1940s for flavoring crab and shrimp.

olive oil   A fragrant liquid produced by crushing or pressing olives. Extra-virgin olive oil—the most flavorful and highest quality—is produced from the first pressing of a batch of olives; oil is also produced from later pressings.

olives   The fruit of the olive tree commonly grown on all sides of the Mediterranean. Black olives are also called ripe olives. Green olives are immature, although they are also widely eaten. *See also* kalmata olives.

oregano   A fragrant, slightly astringent herb used in Greek, Spanish, and Italian dishes.

orzo   A rice-shape pasta used in Greek cooking.

oxidation   The browning of fruit flesh that happens over time and with exposure to air. Oxidation is minimized by rubbing the cut surfaces with a lemon half. Oxidation also affects wine, which is why the taste changes over time after a bottle is opened.

paella   A grand Spanish dish of rice, shellfish, onion, meats, rich broth, and herbs.

pancetta   A type of Italian bacon that's cured, spiced, and dried. It's often flavored with nutmeg, fennel, and garlic.

panko breadcrumbs   A Japanese variety of breadcrumbs that results in a particularly crispy crust when used to coat fried foods.

paprika   A rich, red, warm, earthy spice that also lends a rich, red color to many dishes.

parboil   To partially cook in boiling water or broth, similar to blanching (although blanched foods are quickly cooled with cold water).

pareve   A term used by manufacturers to indicate that a product is primarily dairy free.

Parmesan   A hard, dry, flavorful cheese primarily used grated or shredded as a seasoning for Italian-style dishes.

parsley   A fresh-tasting green, leafy herb, often used as a garnish.

pecans   Rich, buttery nuts, native to North America, that have a high unsaturated fat content.

peppercorns   Large, round, dried berries ground to produce pepper.

pesto   A thick spread or sauce made with fresh basil leaves, garlic, olive oil, pine nuts, and Parmesan cheese. Some newer versions are made with other herbs.

picadillo   A stew or filling usually made from ground beef, popular in Latin American cuisine.

pickle   A food, usually a vegetable such as a cucumber, that's been pickled in brine.

pilaf   A rice dish in which the rice is browned in butter or oil and then cooked in a flavorful liquid such as a broth, often with the addition of meats or vegetables. The rice absorbs the broth, resulting in a savory dish.

pinch   An unscientific measurement term, the amount of an ingredient—typically a dry, granular substance such as an herb or seasoning—you can hold between your finger and thumb.

pine nuts (also **pignoli** or **piñon**)   Nuts grown on pine trees, that are rich (read: high fat), flavorful, and a bit pine-y. Pine nuts are a traditional component of pesto and add a wonderful hearty crunch to many other recipes.

pita bread   A flat, hollow wheat bread often used for sandwiches or sliced, pizza style, into slices. Terrific soft with dips or baked or broiled as a vehicle for other ingredients.

pizza stone   Preheated with the oven, a pizza stone cooks a crust to a delicious, crispy, pizza-parlor texture. It also holds heat well, so a pizza or other food removed from the oven on the stone stay hot for as long as a half hour at the table.

plantain   A relative of the banana, a plantain is larger, milder in flavor, and used as a staple in many Latin American dishes.

poach   To cook a food in simmering liquid, such as water, wine, or broth.

porcini mushrooms   Rich and flavorful mushrooms used in rice and Italian-style dishes.

portobello mushrooms   A mature and larger form of the smaller crimini mushroom, portobellos are brownish, chewy, and flavorful. Often served as whole caps, grilled, and as thin sautéed slices. *See also* crimini mushrooms.

preheat   To turn on an oven, broiler, or other cooking appliance in advance of cooking so the temperature will be at the desired level when the assembled dish is ready for cooking.

prosciutto   Dry, salt-cured ham that originated in Italy.

purée   To reduce a food to a thick, creamy texture, usually using a blender or food processor.

reduce   To boil or simmer a broth or sauce to remove some of the water content, resulting in more concentrated flavor and color.

render   To cook a meat to the point at which its fat melts and can be removed.

reserve   To hold a specified ingredient for another use later in the recipe.

rice vinegar   Vinegar produced from fermented rice or rice wine, popular in Asian-style dishes. Different from rice wine vinegar.

ricotta   A fresh Italian cheese smoother than cottage cheese, with a slightly sweet flavor.

risotto   A popular Italian rice dish made by browning arborio rice in butter or oil and then slowly adding liquid to cook the rice, resulting in a creamy texture.

roast   To cook something uncovered in an oven, usually without additional liquid.

rosemary   A pungent, sweet herb used with chicken, pork, fish, and especially lamb. A little of it goes a long way.

roux   A mixture of butter or another fat and flour, used to thicken sauces and soups.

saffron   A spice made from the stamens of crocus flowers, saffron lends a dramatic yellow color and distinctive flavor to a dish. Use only tiny amounts of this expensive herb.

sage   An herb with a musty yet fruity, lemon-rind scent and "sunny" flavor.

salsa   A style of mixing fresh vegetables and/or fresh fruit in a coarse chop. Salsa can be spicy or not, fruit based or not, and served as a starter on its own (with chips, for example) or as a companion to a main course.

sauté   To pan-cook over lower heat than used for frying.

savory   A popular herb with a fresh, woody taste.

sear   To quickly brown the exterior of a food, especially meat, over high heat to preserve interior moisture.

semolina   The coarsely ground endosperm of durum wheat used in pasta making.

sesame oil   An oil, made from pressing sesame seeds, that's tasteless if clear and aromatic and flavorful if brown.

sesame seeds   Also called "benne," are the crispy nutty seeds of the sesame plant and are used in cooking and baking and are a great source of calcium.

shallot   A member of the onion family that grows in a bulb somewhat like garlic and has a milder onion flavor. When a recipe calls for shallot, use the entire bulb.

shellfish   A broad range of seafood, including clams, mussels, oysters, crabs, shrimp, and lobster. Some people are allergic to shellfish, so take care when including it in recipes.

shiitake mushrooms   Large, dark-brown mushrooms with a hearty, meaty flavor. Can be used either fresh or dried, grilled or as a component in other recipes and as a flavoring source for broth.

short-grain rice   A starchy rice popular for Asian-style dishes because it readily clumps (perfect for eating with chopsticks).

shred   To cut into many long, thin slices.

simmer   To boil gently so the liquid barely bubbles.

skillet (also **frying pan**)   A generally heavy, flat-bottomed metal pan with a handle designed to cook food over heat on a stovetop or campfire.

skim   To remove fat or other material from the top of a liquid.

slice   To cut into thin pieces.

steam   To suspend a food over boiling water and allow the heat of the steam (water vapor) to cook the food. A quick cooking method, steaming preserves the flavor and texture of a food.

steep   To let sit in hot water, as in steeping tea in hot water for 10 minutes.

stew   To slowly cook pieces of food submerged in a liquid. Also a dish that has been prepared by this method.

sticky rice (or **glutinous rice**)   *See* short-grain rice.

Stilton   The famous English blue-veined cheese, delicious with toasted nuts and renowned for its pairing with Port wine.

stir-fry   To cook small pieces of food in a wok or skillet over high heat, moving and turning the food quickly to cook all sides.

stock   A flavorful broth made by cooking meats and/or vegetables with seasonings until the liquid absorbs these flavors. This liquid is then strained and the solids discarded. Can be eaten alone or used as a base for soups and stews.

stone-ground cornmeal   Cornmeal that retains some of the hull and germ of the corn kernel, resulting in more flavor but a shorter shelf life.

strata   A savory bread pudding made with eggs and cheese.

succotash   A cooked vegetable dish usually made of corn and peppers.

tahini   A paste made from sesame seeds, used to flavor many Middle Eastern recipes.

tapenade   A thick, chunky spread made from savory ingredients such as olives, lemon juice, and anchovies.

tarragon   A sweet, rich-smelling herb perfect with seafood, vegetables (especially asparagus), chicken, and pork.

tempeh   A fermented soybean product popular in Indonesia and frequently used in vegetarian cooking. Unlike tofu, the beans stay whole, forming a cake and resulting in higher levels of protein, fiber, nutrients, and flavor.

teriyaki   A Japanese-style sauce composed of soy sauce, rice wine, ginger, and sugar that works well with seafood as well as most meats.

thyme   A minty, zesty herb.

toast   To heat something, usually bread, so it's browned and crisp.

tofu   A cheeselike substance made from soybeans and soy milk.

turmeric   A spicy, pungent yellow root used in many dishes, especially Indian cuisine, for color and flavor. Turmeric is the source of the yellow color in many prepared mustards.

twist   A garnish for an appetizer or other dish, usually made from a lemon or other citrus fruit. To make, cut a thin, $^1/_8$-inch-thick cross-section slice of a lemon or other fruit. Cut from the center of that slice out to the edge on one side. Pull apart the two cut ends in opposite directions.

veal   Meat from a calf, generally characterized by mild flavor and tenderness.

vegan   A person or diet free of all animal products, including dairy.

vegetable steamer   An insert for a large saucepan, or a special pot with tiny holes in the bottom, designed to fit on another pot to hold food to be steamed above boiling water. *See also* steam.

venison   Deer meat.

vinegar   An acidic liquid widely used as dressing and seasoning, often made from fermented grapes, apples, or rice. *See also* balsamic vinegar; cider vinegar; rice vinegar; white vinegar; wine vinegar.

walnuts   A rich, slightly woody-flavored nut.

wasabi   Japanese horseradish, a fiery, pungent condiment used with many Japanese-style dishes. Most often sold as a powder; add water to create a paste.

water chestnuts   A tuber, popular in many types of Asian-style cooking. The flesh is white, crunchy, and juicy, and the vegetable holds its texture whether cool or hot.

whey   A protein found in all dairy products. It's abundant in the liquid remaining when casein is removed from milk and is often dried and added to commercial foods and products.

whisk   To rapidly mix, introducing air to the mixture.

white mushrooms   Button mushrooms. When fresh, they have an earthy smell and an appealing "soft crunch."

white vinegar   The most common type of vinegar, produced from grain.

whole-wheat flour   Wheat flour that contains the entire grain.

wild rice   Actually a grass with a rich, nutty flavor, popular as an unusual and nutritious side dish.

wine vinegar   Vinegar produced from red or white wine.

Worcestershire sauce   Originally developed in India and containing tamarind, this spicy sauce is used as a seasoning for many meats and other dishes.

yeast   Tiny fungi that, when mixed with water, sugar, flour, and heat, release carbon dioxide bubbles, which, in turn, cause the bread to rise.

zest   Small slivers of peel, usually from a citrus fruit such as lemon, lime, or orange.

zester   A kitchen tool used to scrape zest off a fruit. A small grater also works well.

Further Resources

Whether you're hunting down dairy-free ingredients or seeking a specialist to help you determine your own dairy-free goals, this appendix will prove a valuable starting point. From online shops and professional organizations to websites and recommendations for further reading, the resources that follow provide the information you need to dig a little deeper into the dairy-free way of life.

Products

Many more dairy-free and vegan products are now available at local super-markets as well as health food stores, as awareness of milk allergy and lactose intolerance has increased. Online shopping sources continue to be valuable for hard-to-find products. Here are several excellent websites where you can order what you need:

Cosmo's Vegan Shoppe
www.cosmosveganshoppe.com
This is a reliable source for nutritional yeast flakes and dairy-free beverages such as oat and rice milk.

Vegan Essentials
www.veganessentials.com
Vegan Essentials has an excellent array of both perishable and pantry items, including cheese substitutes and chocolate.

The Vegan Store

www.veganstore.com

This is one of the best dairy-free sources for "cheese" and "sour cream," all cold-packed for safe shipping.

The Vegetarian Express

www.thevegetarianexpress.com

This store boasts a downloadable catalog and an impressive array of seasonings and gravy mixes.

Organizations

Important government and professional organizations exist to assist families dealing with milk allergy as well as other food allergies. You'll find detailed information, contact sources, and helpful referrals from the following agencies and institutes.

The American Academy of Allergy, Asthma and Immunology

www.aaaai.org

The American College of Allergy, Asthma and Immunology

www.acaai.org

These professional organizations have public information resources for allergies and food allergies. In addition, they offer search engines to locate Board-certified allergists by entering your zip code and specific interests.

The American Academy of Pediatrics

www.aap.org

This is the professional organization for U.S. pediatricians. The site includes information for parents on a variety of health topics, including allergies.

Asthma and Allergy Foundation of America

www.aafa.org

This organization offers numerous resources for people with all types of allergic problems.

The Center for Food Safety and Applied Nutrition

www.cfsan.fda.gov

This division of the U.S. Food and Drug Association assists with matters of public health and policy regarding food safety, including allergies. Information about labeling and other food allergy issues is posted here. The site also includes links for reporting problems with foods (for example, undeclared allergens) through www.fda.gov/medwatch.

The Food Allergy and Anaphylaxis Network

www.foodallergy.org

This major resource for individuals and families with food allergies provides parent educational conferences and educational books and videos. Comprehensive programs for preschools, schools, and camps are available, as are books for children and teens, research updates, and much more.

The Food Allergy Initiative

www.foodallergyinitiative.org

This organization's mission includes raising funds for and increasing public awareness of food allergy research efforts, and championing improved safety.

The Jaffe Food Allergy Institute at Mount Sinai

www.mssm.edu/jaffe_food_allergy

Located in Manhattan, Mount Sinai School of Medicine is internationally recognized for ground-breaking clinical and basic-science research on food allergies.

MedicAlert

www.medicalert.org

This nonprofit organization offers jewelry that provides medical information about the wearer.

Websites

Numerous websites and blogs abound where dairy-free folks and parents of children with milk allergy can gather and discuss a variety of issues. Although they're mostly specific to allergies, many also address lactose intolerance and other food allergies.

About.com: Dairy-Free Cooking

www.dairyfreecooking.about.com

This site is loaded with enticing dairy-free recipes, many also vegan, and provides a good discussion on substituting for dairy products in baking.

Avoiding Milk Protein

www.avoidingmilkprotein.com

Created by a dairy-free mom, this site includes a blog with valuable informational links.

Go Dairy Free

www.godairyfree.org

A companion site to the *Go Dairy Free Guide* by Alisa Marie Fleming, this is probably the most comprehensive and valuable source online for learning everything there is to know about dairy-free living for families.

Got No Milk

www.gotnomilk.wordpress.com

Here, a lactose-intolerant blogger shares mouth-watering recipes and luscious pictures of her creations.

No Whey, Mama

www.nowheymama.blogspot.com

Fun to read with great photos, this blog created by a dairy-free mom has lots of tips for families, as well as kid-friendly recipes.

Further Reading

Whether you'd like to learn how to make your own dairy-free cheese or explore other food allergies in depth, numerous books can help you on your journey.

Coss, Linda Marienhoff. *How to Manage Your Child's Life-Threatening Food Allergies: Practical Tips for Everyday Life.* Lake Forest, CA: Plumtree Press, 2004.

Fleming, Alisa Marie. *Go Dairy Free: The Guide and Cookbook for Milk Allergies, Lactose Intolerance, and Casein-Free Living.* Henderson, NV: Fleming Ink, 2008.

Jardine, Denise. *Recipes for Dairy-Free Living.* Berkeley, CA: Celestial Arts, 2002.

Kidder, Beth. *The Milk-Free Kitchen: Living Well Without Dairy Products.* New York, NY: Holt Paperbacks, 1991.

Pascal, Cybele. *The Whole Foods Allergy Cookbook.* Ridgefield, CT: Vital Health Publishing, 2005.

Rogers, Jeff. *Vice Cream: Over 70 Sinfully Delicious Dairy-Free Delights.* Berkeley, CA: Ten Speed Press, 2004.

Sicherer, Scott H., M.D. *Understanding and Managing Your Child's Food Allergies.* Baltimore, MD: John Hopkins University Press, 2006.

Stepaniak, Jo. *The Ultimate Uncheese Cookbook: Delicious Dairy-Free Cheeses, and Classic "Uncheese" Dishes.* Summertown, TN: Book Publishing Company (TN), 2003.

Vezzani, Juventa. *The Milk Allergy Companion and Cookbook.* Charleston, SC: BookSurge Publishing, 2009.

Zukin, Jane. *Dairy-Free Cookbook: Over 250 Recipes for People with Lactose Intolerance or Milk Allergy.* New York, NY: Three Rivers Press, 1998.

Decoding Infant Formula

Breast milk is the drink of choice for infants, but for infants who are supplemented or weaned, a number of commercial infant formulas are available. These formulas are nutritionally "complete," meaning they're nutritionally balanced as a sole source of nutrition for newborns and infants, and offer essential dietary nutrients not available in, for example, whole milk, soy, or rice drinks, which would not be a good choice for infants. Which formula you use depends on your baby's needs. Discuss your options with your pediatrician, especially if your infant was born premature.

Here are some types of infant formulas (with a few brand names as examples):

Milk-based infant formula (Enfamil/Mead Johnson Nutritionals, Similac/Ross Products)   These formulas are based on cow's milk and contain cow's milk proteins, including casein and whey, in their natural state. An infant with a cow's milk allergy would likely have an allergic reaction to this type of infant formula.

Extensively hydrolyzed casein (Enfamil Nutramigen Lipil/Mead Johnson Nutritionals, Enfamil Pregestimil/Mead Johnson Nutritionals, Similac Alimentum Advance/Ross Products)   These formulas are processed in a way that breaks down the cow's milk proteins "extensively," somewhat like being predigested. More than 90 percent of infants with a cow's milk allergy tolerate this formula. This formula, when compared to whole cow's milk protein formula, has allergy-prevention effects.

Partially hydrolyzed whey (Good Start Supreme/Nestlé USA)   This formula is based on one of the types of cow's milk protein, the whey proteins, and is processed to break down the protein "partially." An infant with milk allergy would likely have an allergic reaction to this type of formula. Partially hydrolyzed whey formula has been studied for allergy prevention in at-risk children, and is effective compared to cow's milk formula and almost as effective as the extensive hydrolysate.

Partially hydrolyzed whey/casein (Enfamil Gentlease Lipil/Mead Johnson Nutritionals)   This formula has both of the cow's milk proteins partially "digested." It has not been studied for allergy prevention. It would likely cause an allergic reaction in an infant with a milk allergy.

Soy (Similac Isomil, Enfamil ProSobee)   Soy formulas are not based on any mammalian milk proteins, but rather on proteins from soybeans. There is a 10 to 14 percent chance that an infant with sudden allergic reactions to milk would also be allergic to soy, and about a 50 percent chance that an infant with chronic allergic gut problems from cow's milk would react to soy. Therefore, soy is usually not recommended to treat milk allergies. Soy formula is not considered to "prevent" allergy compared to milk-based infant formulas. A soy formula might be chosen for personal preference to avoid animal products, to avoid having lactose (milk sugar), although lactose intolerance is rare in infants, except briefly after certain viral infections, or for infants with some types of medical conditions that require avoiding milk sugars.

Partially hydrolyzed soy (Good Start Supreme Soy/Nestlé USA)   This formula is similar to the whole soy protein formula, except that the soy proteins are partially processed (predigested). It has not been studied for the prevention of allergy.

Free amino acid–based (Neocate/Nutricia North America, Gaithersburg, MD, EleCare/Ross Pediatrics)   This type of formula is not made from animal or vegetable protein, but rather uses amino acids, the building blocks of proteins. Children with allergies are extremely unlikely to be allergic to this type of formula, and even a child who is allergic to extensively hydrolyzed casein-based formula should tolerate this formula. The formula has not been studied for prevention effects.

Index

E

F

G

H

I–J

S

U–V

W-X-Y-Z

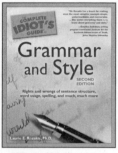
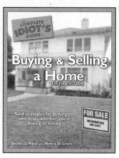
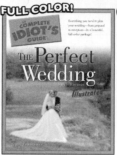
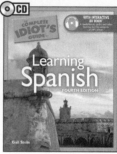
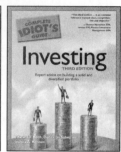
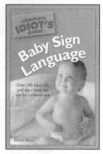
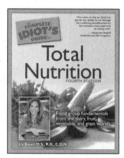
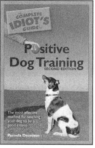
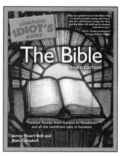
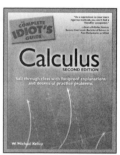
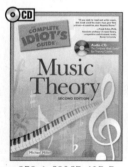
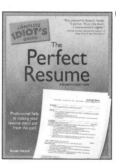
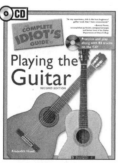
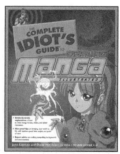
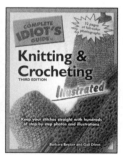